ABNORMAL HEART RHYTHMS

Edited by **Francisco R. Breijo-Marquez**

Abnormal Heart Rhythms
http://dx.doi.org/10.5772/59212
Edited by Francisco R. Breijo-Marquez

Contributors

José Joaquín Rieta, Raúl Alcaraz, Fereshteh Mehraein, Bernhard Schaller, Toshiya Kurotobi, Paul Gould, Lucie Riedlbauchova

Published by InTech

Janeza Trdine 9, 51000 Rijeka, Croatia

Publishing Process Manager Ivona Lovric

Technical Editor InTech DTP team

Cover InTech Design team

First published August, 2015

Printed in Croatia

Additional hard copies can be obtained from orders@intechopen.com

Abnormal Heart Rhythms, Edited by Francisco R. Breijo-Marquez

p. cm.

ISBN 978-953-51-2148-0

For EU product safety concerns:
IN TECH d.o.o., Prolaz Marije Krucifikse Kozulić 3, 51000 Rijeka, Croatia,
info@intechopen.com or visit our website at intechopen.com.

Meet the editor

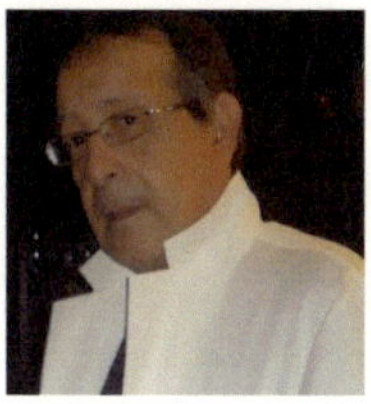

Prof. Breijo-Marquez is a professor of Clinical and Experimental Cardiology. He is also a research director at East Boston University (on voluntary leave), Hartford University (on voluntary leave), Murcia University, and C.S. Abanilla (currently). He is the director of Doctoral Theses on Clinical and Experimental Cardiology, Education and Research of Heart. Prof. Breijo-Marquez is an advisor, an editorial board Member, and a reviewer of several scientific committees from several institutions and specialized journals. He has published several textbooks, clinical works, and clinical trials in his research field. Currently, he works as a research director in his institutions.

Contents

Preface

By reading this book, the reader can get more knowledge on some of the most common cardiac arrhythmias.

Electrical disturbances in the atria of the heart have been very well presented in this book by different authors. The main chapters of the book refer to such supraventricular arrhythmias.

Interested readers on this topic can value the different antiarrhythmic agents against such cardiac arrhythmias, mainly the role of "Amiodarone" in these kinds of cardiac events.

This is definitely an interesting book, and it is worthy of being read.

My congratulations to all authors who have written the different chapters covering some of the most interesting advances on this topic.

Their dedication is appreciated.

Francisco R. Breijo-Marquez, FR, PhD
East Boston Hospital, School of Medicine,
02136 Tremont St., Boston, MA, USA

Section 1

Atrial Electrical Disorders

Chapter 1

Atrial Flutter — Diagnosis, Management and Treatment

Shameer Ahmed, Andrew Claughton and
Paul A. Gould

Additional information is available at the end of the chapter

http://dx.doi.org/10.5772/60700

Abstract

Atrial flutter and atrial fibrillation are the two most common arrhythmias which originate in the atrium and cause a narrow complex tachycardia which has thromboembolic risk and coexist clinically. Atrial flutter has been traditionally defined as a supraventricular arrhythmia with an atrial rate of 240–360 beats per minute (bpm). It is due to a macro-reentrant atrial activation around an anatomical barrier. Atrial flutter can be described as typical and atypical. Due to recent innovations in technology, catheter ablation has emerged as the most viable option with a success rate of more than 90 %. Three-dimensional electroanatomical mapping is useful in the treatment of atypical atrial flutter.

Keywords: Typical atrial flutter, Atypical atrial flutter, Cavo-tricuspid isthmus (CTI), Radio-frequency ablation (RFA), Differential pacing, Bidirectional block, Mapping, Entrainment

1. Introduction

Atrial arrhythmias are significant contributors for cardiac co-morbidity especially for stroke, heart failure and recurrent hospitalisations. The more frequent clinically encountered atrial tachyarrhythmias include atrial tachycardia, atrial flutter and atrial fibrillation. Although they are supraventricular in origin, apart from atrial tachycardia, they are not generally included in the nomenclature of supraventricular tachycardia. Atrial flutter has been traditionally defined as a macro-reentrant arrhythmia around a macroscopic (more than 2 cm in area) anatomical barrier that is confined within the atria. The atrial rate in atrial flutter is approximately 240–360 beats per minute (bpm) with no distinct isoelectric period between the flutter 'F' waves. It is generally paroxysmal in nature in a structurally healthy heart. If the tachycardia persists for a prolonged period, it frequently can degenerate into atrial fibrillation, particularly if the patient already has structural heart disease. As such, atrial flutter and atrial fibrillation often coexist.

Atrial tachycardia is typically characterised by atrial rates >100 bpm but less than 240 bpm with discrete activation sequences and non-sinus P waves including a baseline isoelectric period between these waves on ECG. Its mechanism can be due to triggered activity or increased automaticity of atrial cells. These mechanisms are distinct from that of atrial flutter which is macro-reentrant; however, atrial tachycardia can also be re-entrant in mechanism similar to atrial flutter but on a microscopic level (re-entry around barriers of less than 2 cm).

Atrial fibrillation is due to fibrillatory waves in the atria with rates that are typically greater than 300 bpm in the atria. Currently these waves are considered chaotic and do not behave like the macro-reentry wavefront of atrial flutter. Re-entry however is still thought to play a role in atrial fibrillation, but its exact involvement is unknown.

In this chapter, we will discuss the classification, pathophysiology, clinical presentation, electrocardiographic characteristics, electrophysiological testing and both the pharmacological and ablative management of atrial flutter.

2. Epidemiology

Evidence based on epidemiological studies in the USA suggests that the overall incidence of atrial flutter is about 88/100,000 person-years. When adjusted for age, the incidence of atrial flutter in men is more than 2.5 times that of women. The age-specific incidence of atrial flutter increases exponentially with age from 5/100,000 person-years in those less than 50 years old to 587/100,000 person-years among individuals more than 80 years [1].

The risk factors that are identified as the highest risk for developing atrial flutter include male gender, increasing age, heart failure, chronic obstructive pulmonary disease (COPD) and diabetes mellitus.

3. Classification

Classification for atrial flutter can be based on electrocardiography (ECG) or anatomical and electrophysiological mechanisms [2].

Originally, atrial flutter was classified as types I and II [3]. Type I atrial flutter is the designated classical sawtooth-appearing atrial tachycardia with rate >240 to 360 bpm, lacking an isoelectric baseline between deflections (i.e. continuous flutter wave). Type II atrial flutter was defined on the basis of a rapid rate (>350 bpm) and the inability to be entrained. However, there are no further systematic electrophysiological studies of type II atrial flutter, and the mechanism is unknown. Now, atrial flutter is referred to as being either typical or atypical.

For clinical and practical purposes, atrial flutter can be broadly classified as per Table 1.

Cavo-tricuspid isthmus (CTI)-dependent atrial flutter or typical flutter	**Non-CTI-dependent atrial flutters or atypical atrial flutters**
Typical atrial flutter (counterclockwise right atrial flutter)	Right atrial free wall
Clockwise or reverse typical right atrial flutter	Upper-loop re-entry
	Lower-loop re-entry
	Left atrial flutter, including mitral annular atrial flutter, scar and pulmonary vein-dependent atrial flutter and coronary sinus atrial flutter, left septal atrial flutter

Table 1. Classification of atrial flutter

In 2001, the European Society of Cardiology and the North American Society of Pacing and Electrophysiology proposed a classification [4] that takes into consideration both anatomic features and electrophysiological mechanisms.

3.1. Typical atrial flutter (Counterclockwise CTI-Dependant right atrial macro-reentry)

Counterclockwise re-entry is the most common type of macro-reentrant atrial tachycardia. The anatomical boundaries for this re-entrant tachycardia are anteriorly the tricuspid orifice and posteriorly the orifices of vena cavae and the eustachian ridge and the region of the crista terminalis [5, 6]. The conduction of macro-reentrant circuit is up the inter-atrial septum and around the roof towards the crista terminalis and then down the anterolateral wall (RA free wall anterior to the crista terminalis) to the lateral aspect of the tricuspid annulus (Figure 2).

3.2. Reverse typical atrial flutter (Clockwise right atrial macro-reentry)

A reverse direction of rotation of the above circuit in the right atrium (i.e. ascending the lateral wall and descending the posterior and septal walls; see Figure 2) can occur clinically in the typical atrial flutter circuit in 10 % of cases [7]. This is still called typical atrial flutter because the re-entry path is the same, even though the direction of activation is reversed. Reverse typical atrial flutter has also been called clockwise atrial flutter, referring to the direction of endocardial activation from a left anterior oblique fluoroscopic perspective. It is proposed that there is a 9:1 clinical predominance of typical (counterclockwise) atrial flutter compared to clockwise re-entry. This may be related to the localisation of an area with a low safety factor for conduction in the atrial flutter isthmus, close to the atrial septum.

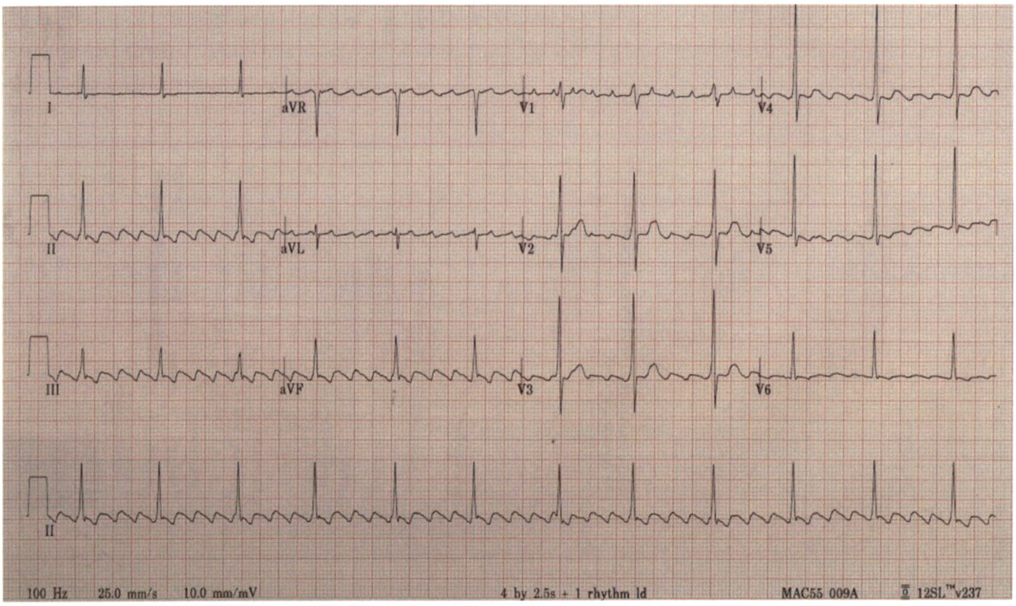

Figure 1. ECG of counterclockwise CTI-dependant atrial flutter: Flutter waves are continuous without an isoelectric baseline, best seen in the inferior leads. The 'F waves' (Flutter waves) are most commonly conducted in the ventricle in a 2:1 manner, giving a regular ventricular response during the arrhythmia typically 150 beats per minute (bpm); however, other multiples of conduction can occur such as 3:1 or 4:1 (Figure 1), giving slow ventricular rates during the arrhythmia. Less commonly, irregular rhythms can be encountered with a variable pattern in conduction to the ventricle

3.3. Lower-Loop Re-entry

Counterclockwise re-entry around the inferior vena cava (see Figures 2 and 12) where the anterior arm of the circuit is the inferior vena cava. The posterior arm is the low posterior right atrial wall with conduction across the crista terminalis [8]. Electroanatomical or conventional mapping shows activation rotating around areas of low-voltage electrograms in the right atrial free wall, not due to surgical scars.

3.4. Atypical atrial flutter

3.4.1. Lesion macro-reentrant atrial tachycardia

In this macro-reentrant atrial tachycardia, the central obstacle of the circuit is an atriotomy scar, a septal prosthetic patch, a suture line or a line of fixed block secondary to radio-frequency ablation or other causes of scar [9]. This can also lead to complicated tracts for the re-entry circuit.

3.4.2. Right atrial free (Lateral) wall atriotomy tachycardia

The best characterisation of atriotomy macro-reentrant atrial tachycardia is due to activation around an area of low voltage or scar in the lateral right atrial wall, with a main superoinferior axis.

http://dx.doi.org/10.5772/60700

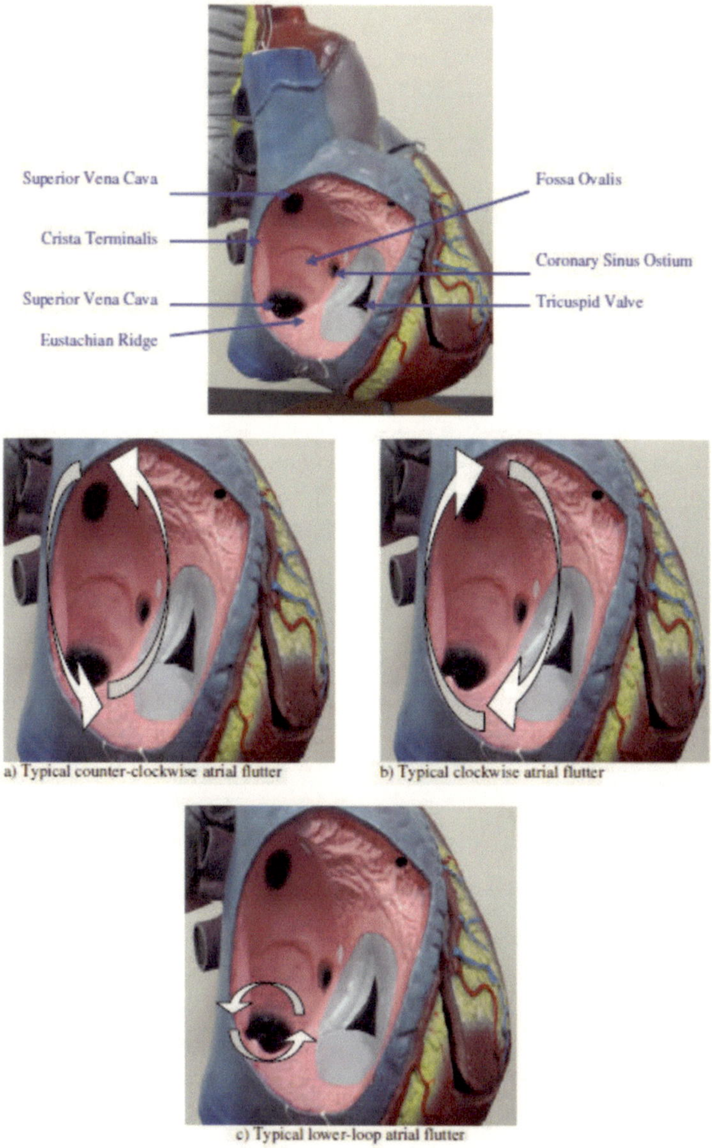

Figure 2. Typical Atrial flutter

3.5. Double-wave re-entry

In this macro-reentrant tachycardia, two wavefronts circulate simultaneously in the same re-entrant circuit. A stable macro-reentrant atrial tachycardia can originate in the left atrium. The clinical incidence is not well known but may be 1/10th that of typical atrial flutter. There is still little information on the anatomical bases of left atrial macro-reentry tachycardia, although recent reports have characterised the substrate as showing wide scarred areas with low voltage or absent electrograms [10].

4. Clinical presentation

Atrial flutter can be paroxysmal or persistent. When atrial flutter is associated with an increased ventricular response, it can result in palpitations, shortness of breath, chest pain, fatigue or pre-syncope. If a patient presents with atrial flutter and a rapid ventricular rate, stroke, tachycardia-induced cardiomyopathy and rarely myocardial infarction are complications that can be encountered. Syncope in the setting of atrial flutter is rare if there is no significant cardiac history [11]. When presenting because of a more prolonged episode, increased symptoms of heart failure may be evident. Occasionally, atrial flutter is an incidental finding on ECG with patients who are completely asymptomatic.

5. Management

Therapy for atrial flutter has two goals: management of the arrhythmia itself with either rate control or rhythm control and management of the complications of the arrhythmia with stroke prophylaxis [12].

5.1. Non-invasive management

5.1.1. Rate control

Rate control is generally reserved for patients who are in permanent atrial flutter and have no or minimal symptoms and cannot achieve rhythm control due to co-morbidities or are not willing to undergo procedures or take medications. There is debate in the literature about what exactly is adequate rate control; this however pertains to atrial fibrillation as it has not been specifically studied in atrial flutter. The same parameters however could generally be applied as the goal is to avoid tachycardia-induced cardiomyopathy whilst preserving exercise capacity. Typically, the aim is an average 24-hour heart rate over 24 hours of 80 bpm and a maximum of less than 130 bpm [13]. An emerging data however shows that less strict control such as heart rates less than an average 24-hour heart rate of less than 110 bpm is adequate [13, 14]. Various pharmacological agents which are used in non-invasive management are presented in Table 2.

Rate control of atrial flutter can be very difficult to achieve pharmacologically. It is important to understand that atrial flutter ablation has a high success rate unlike atrial fibrillation, and extreme methods of rate control such as pacemaker implantation and AV nodal ablation are rarely used as a management strategy.

Rate control	Rhythm control	Stroke prophylaxis
Beta-blocker	Class Ia: procainamide	Coumadin
Calcium channel blockers	Class Ic: flecainide, propafenone	Newer anticoagulation agents: dabigatran
Digoxin	Class III: sotalol, amiodarone, ibutilide,	Rivaroxaban
Amiodarone	dofetilide	Apixaban

Table 2. Pharmacological management therapies

5.1.2. Rhythm control

In an acute setting, atrial flutter with hemodynamic compromise or rarely significant cardiac symptoms (i.e. severe chest pain), synchronised direct current cardioversion is indicated to revert patients to sinus rhythm. Previously, lower defibrillator outputs such as 50 J were employed to prevent pain, but the current recommendation is 200 J biphasic with either anteroposterior or midline and lateral defibrillation pad positioning. There is no difference in pain and potential of ventricular fibrillation induction with lower energy levels.

In clinically stable atrial flutter, the various non-invasive management therapies include cardioversion (electrical or pharmacological) and rate control with pharmacotherapy to slow down AV nodal conduction (see Table 2) or if an atrial pacing lead is in situ rapid atrial pacing for overdrive termination. This is commonly burst pacing to depolarise tissue in the macro-reentrant circuit into which the activation front of the arrhythmia is depolarising to terminate the tachycardia. The pacing is typically for three to five seconds at rate approximately 20 ms less than flutter wave cycle length; though this also has the potential to cause atrial fibrillation.

For a list of antiarrhythmic drugs for cardioversion of atrial flutter, refer to Table 2. Classes Ia and Ic can result in slowing the rate of atrial flutter which can facilitate 1:1 conduction of atrial flutter via AV node and cause a rapid ventricular rate. Thus, it is recommended to have concurrent AV blocking agents to control the ventricular response. These antiarrhythmic agents are not very well studied in atrial flutter patient population. The data about their efficacy is derived from clinical trials where atrial flutter was grouped with atrial fibrillation. In terms of prevention of atrial flutter recurrence, flecainide and dofetilide have a long-term efficacy of 50 % and 70 %, respectively [15, 16].

5.2. Stroke prevention

Anticoagulation is key to preventing ischemic cerebrovascular events [17]. It is extremely important when either above-mentioned management option is considered. Even though the evidence for anticoagulation in the atrial flutter patient population is not as robust as for atrial fibrillation, it is felt that the risks are similar especially for typical cavo-tricuspid isthmus-dependent atrial flutter. Thromboembolic prophylaxis is indicated in the management of chronic atrial flutter similar to atrial fibrillation. In our clinical practice, we use CHA2DS-VASc score which has superseded the older CHADS2 score to calculate the annual risk of cerebral thromboembolic event [18]. For oral anticoagulants that are used to prevent stroke, refer to Table 2. Patients who have atrial flutter and undergo DC cardioversion should be on novel anticoagulation or on warfarin with therapeutic international normalised ratio (INR) (>2) for a minimum period of three weeks prior to the DCCV and for a minimum of one month later. The new oral anticoagulants do not have as much data for direct-current cardioversion as warfarin therapy, and some clinicians perform trans-oesophageal echocardiograph prior to direct-current cardioversion [19]. There is no role for aspirin in stroke prophylaxis as the risks of bleeding are greater than the benefit of stroke reduction.

5.3. Invasive strategy

5.3.1. Typical cavo-tricuspid-dependent atrial flutter

A standard electrophysiological (EP) case for typical CTI-dependent atrial flutter most often requires the use of three catheters; these include the ablation catheter, a multipolar coronary sinus catheter and a right atrial (RA) mapping catheter. The RA mapping catheter can be either a decapolar or duodecapolar catheter (sometimes referred to as orbital catheter) and is placed along the lateral RA wall anterior to the crista terminalis with the tip down to the lateral inferior RA and tricuspid annulus. Some operators also prefer to additionally use a His and/or right ventricular catheter (Figure 3). Radio-frequency ablation (RFA) is the most commonly used ablation modality in treatment of atrial flutter.

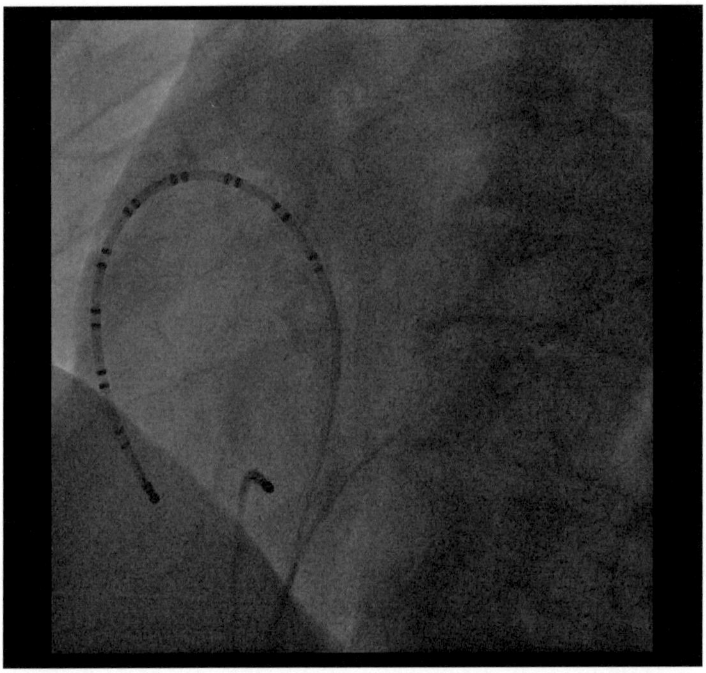

Figure 3. Fluoroscopic image of catheters used for a typical atrial flutter study with duodecapolar catheter in the right atrium, ablation catheter at the cavo-tricuspid isthmus and decapolar catheter in the coronary sinus (courtesy of PA hospital EP Lab)

http://dx.doi.org/10.5772/60700

A similar catheter configuration may be used for an atypical or non-CTI-dependent atrial flutter although a 3D mapping system for these arrhythmias is highly beneficial and can negate the need for other electrogram-based mapping catheters. The mapping system can be utilised to define the entire macro-reentrant circuit by identifying the anatomical boundaries and the ablation target which is generally the area of slow conduction. A line of block is achieved by making a linear ablation line between areas of conduction block (discussed under Radio-Frequency Ablation).

5.4. Electrophysiological study

Generally with cavo-tricuspid isthmus-dependent ablation, there is little electrophysiological study performed as the target of ablation and arrhythmia circuit are known. However, manoeuvres such as entrainment (discussed below) can still be used to confirm cavo-tricuspid isthmus dependence. In atypical atrial flutter ablation, entrainment manoeuvres can be used to localise the arrhythmia circuit. However, with the advent of non-fluoroscopic mapping, entrainment is being employed less frequently to confirm isthmus dependence.

Entrainment is used to determine if a specific anatomical site is a part of the re-entrant circuit [20]. To confirm that atrial flutter is typical and cavo-tricuspid isthmus dependant (not a bystander), entrainment from the CTI and/or another site such as the proximal coronary sinus is performed. By entraining in the atria at a cycle length approximately 10 to 20 ms faster than the tachycardia cycle length and then measuring the post-pacing interval (PPI) (return cycle length), one can determine if CTI (or pacing site) is a part of the re-entrant circuit (Figures 4). The post-pacing interval is the time between the last pacing stimulus that entrained the tachycardia and the next recorded electrogram at the pacing site. The pacing site is considered to be a part of the circuit if the post-pacing interval (PPI) is equal or within 30 ms of tachycardia cycle length.

If entrainment from the isthmus does not demonstrate isthmus involvement, further thought needs to be carried out regarding treatment options, as the tachycardia is likely to be atypical and 3D mapping may be more appropriate.

5.5. Radio-Frequency Ablation (RFA)

Ablation therapy for typical atrial flutter targets the cavo-tricuspid isthmus (CTI). It is a narrow point of the circuit and the slow conduction part of the circuit between two nonconductive boundaries; anteriorly this is bounded by the tricuspid annulus and posteriorly by IVC. It is easily accessible percutaneously and distant from the AV node. Conventionally, atrial flutter ablation involved delivering RF energy in a linear ablative line across the entire isthmus to create bidirectional block. Ablation is started on or near the tricuspid annulus and the catheter brought (dragged) back along the isthmus towards the IVC. Ablation can be performed in both atrial flutter and during atrial pacing (empirically) from the coronary sinus but can equally be performed with pacing from the lower right atrium.

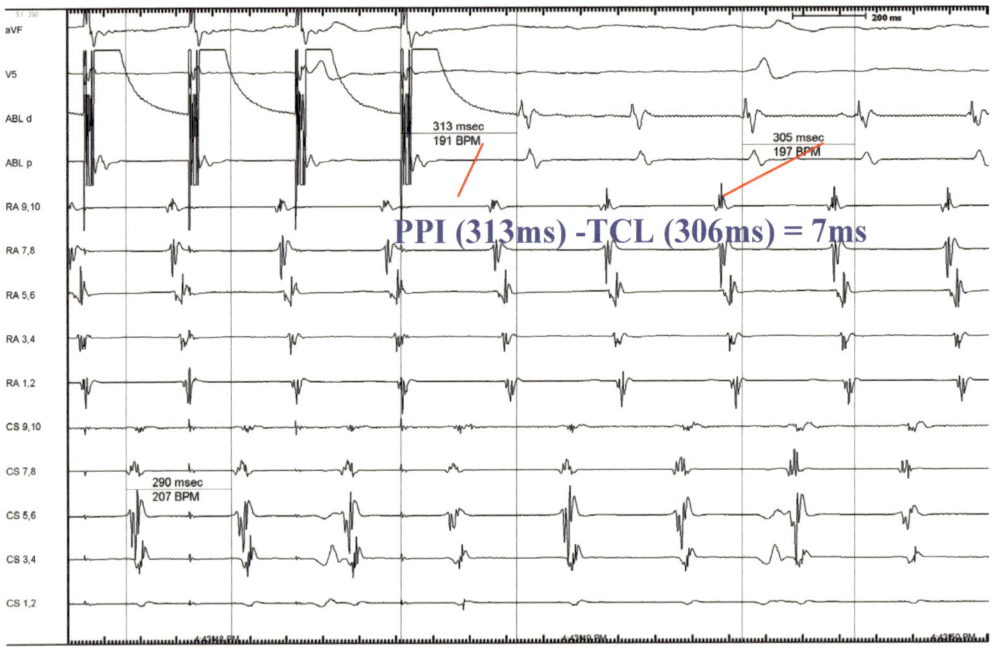

Figure 4. Entrainment of typical CTI ablation demonstrating that pacing site (ablation catheter) is within the circuit of the tachycardia. PPI – TCL = 7 ms. Note also the unidirectional activation of the lateral RA wall superiorly (RA 9,10) to inferiorly (RA 1,2) (courtesy of PAH EP Lab)

6. Post-ablation bidirectional electrophysiological study

6.1. Bidirectional block

This is the electrophysiological endpoint of ablation of the isthmus in CTI-dependent atrial flutter [21]. Activation mapping to measure the trans-isthmus conduction time, differential pacing and online double potentials are the three commonly used techniques that can be employed to determine if the ablation has been successful and bidirectional block has been achieved.

6.2. Activation mapping

Activation mapping involves pacing from either side of the ablation line (proximal CS pacing low lateral RA are commonly used). With incomplete CTI ablation, the wavefront along the RA mapping catheter will be fused as conducts in different directions as depicted in Figure 5 and 6.

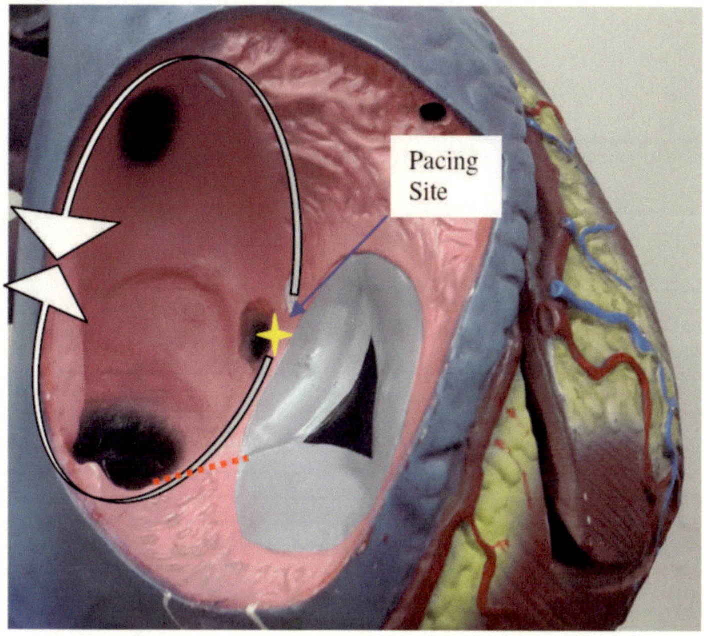

Figure 5. Pacing site from proximal coronary sinus.

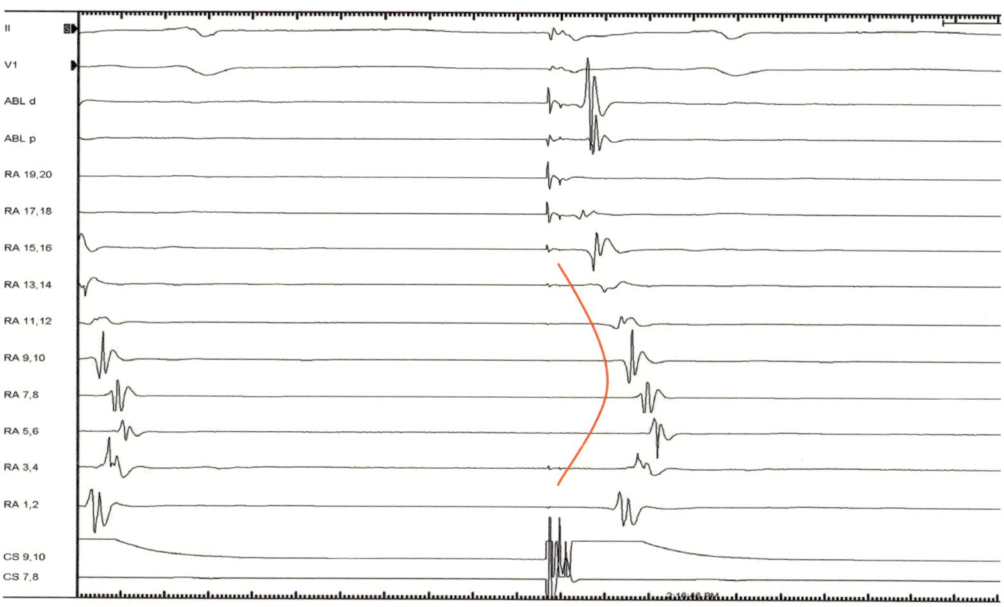

Figure 6. Prior to CTI ablation depicting activation pattern in the right atrium. It is chevron shaped due to persistent conduction through the isthmus and fusion of wavefront in the right atrium

With successful bidirectional block, the activation along the RA catheter is uniform (Figures 7 and 8).

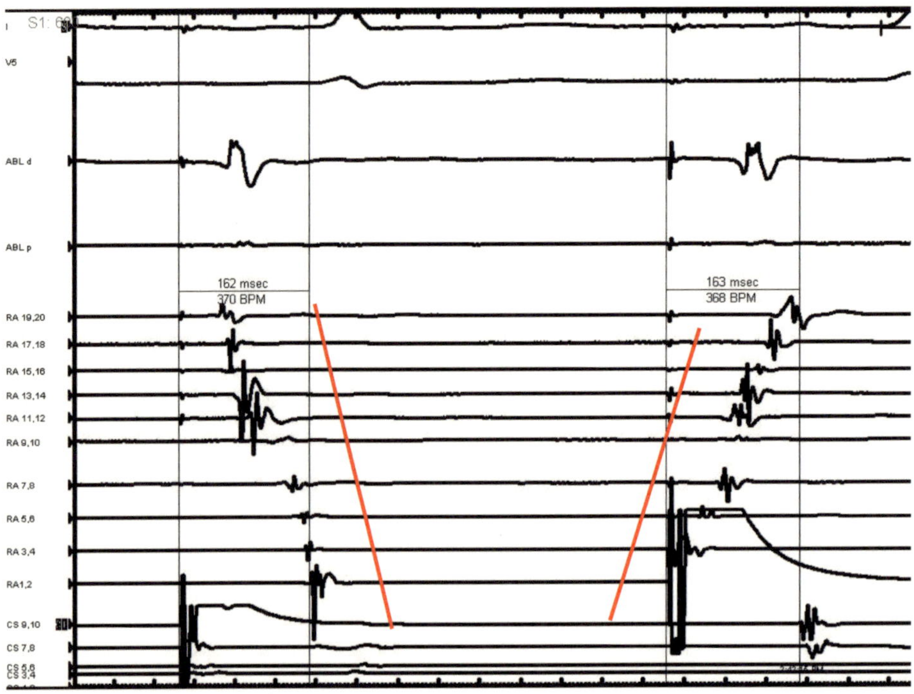

Figure 7. Bidirectional block demonstrated by activation; A, indicates proximal CS pacing and sequential activation around the RA from proximal to distal RA catheter; B, pacing from distal RA with sequential activation from distal to proximal RA – both showing conduction block over the cavo-tricuspid isthmus region (Courtesy of PAH EP Lab)

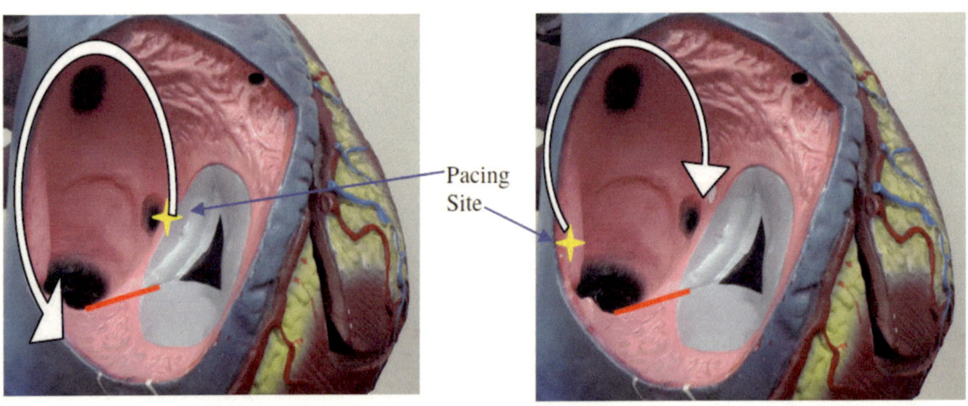

Figure 8. Pacing from proximal sinus and from RA lateral/anterior wall respectively

http://dx.doi.org/10.5772/60700

6.3. Trans-isthmus conduction time

During the flutter circuit, the isthmus conduction time accounts for ~33 % of the cycle time, and the RA cycle accounts for ~66 % of the cycle length [22]. The isthmus conduction time is measured from the pacing site to the signal arising on the other side of the cavo-tricuspid isthmus.

At baseline, if the patient is in sinus rhythm, pacing from proximal CS, the measurement would be to low in RA and vice versa. When there is no damage to the isthmus, conduction time should be <90 ms. Post-successful CTI ablation trans-isthmus conduction time increases by 50 % [23] or from <90 ms to >140 ms.

6.4. Differential pacing

One important manoeuvre to establish bidirectional block is to perform differential pacing [24]. Differential pacing is most useful when there is a very slow conduction across CTI with long conduction time, leaving it difficult to confirm bidirectional block with trans-isthmus time measurements and activation mapping. It involves pacing at two different sites on the lateral side of the CTI line (along the lateral wall of the RA).

During differential pacing, the wavefront conducts in two directions, counterclockwise towards the isthmus line and clockwise around the right atria towards the septal border of the CTI line (or the CS ostium). When isthmus block has been achieved, moving the catheter further away from the CTI line should result in a decreased clockwise activation time from lateral pacing site to the CS ostium. It can also be performed the other way by pacing from a standard site (CS ostium) and then positioning the mapping catheter in two sites on the lateral side of the CTI line.

6.5. Online double potentials

Online double potentials represent an area of local conduction block at the line of ablation. A 110 ms separation of signals has been identified as a 100 % positive predictor value for isthmus block [25]. The early first signal results from the initial wavefront from the pacing stimulus reaching the line, which then encounters block. The second delayed signal results from activation entering the opposite side of the line of ablation.

The online double potential technique is an assistance guide to determining bidirectional block and should be used in conjunction with other methods.

6.6. Atypical atrial flutter

An isthmus for atypical flutter can be formed by a number of anatomical barriers, including the tricuspid or mitral annuluses, superior or inferior vena cava, pulmonary veins or the CS ostium. It can also form a circuit secondary to scars which can occur after infarction, myocarditis or congenital or valvular surgery. Electrically, the isthmus can be represented by low amplitude or fractionated signals, areas of slow conduction and/or double potentials. Double

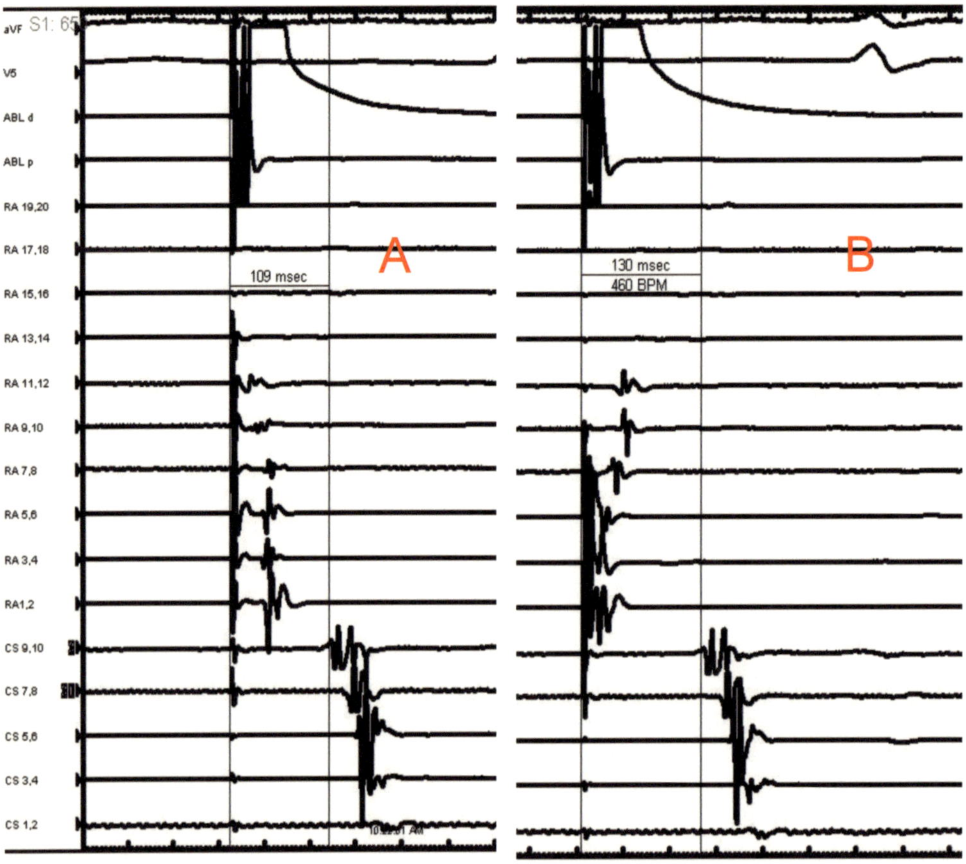

Figure 9. Differential pacing with pacing from RA 11, 12 of a duodecapolar catheter (lateral) and then more laterally from site RA 3,4 of the duodecapolar catheter (courtesy of PA EP Lab)

potential indicates line of block and fragmented potentials and mid-diastolic potentials indicate critical zones of slow conduction.

Atypical atrial flutter can be very difficult to assess and treat. The use of anatomical and 3D mapping systems has an important role in identification and successful ablation of atypical atrial flutter.

6.7. 2D mapping and electrophysiology

To assist with 2D and signal mapping, it is very important to know the chamber the flutter is originating from.

6.7.1. Localising atypical flutter to the right atrium

Activation of the coronary sinus from proximal to distal is the first clue that the flutter is most likely to be originating from the RA. Other clues include RA activation time accounting for

http://dx.doi.org/10.5772/60700

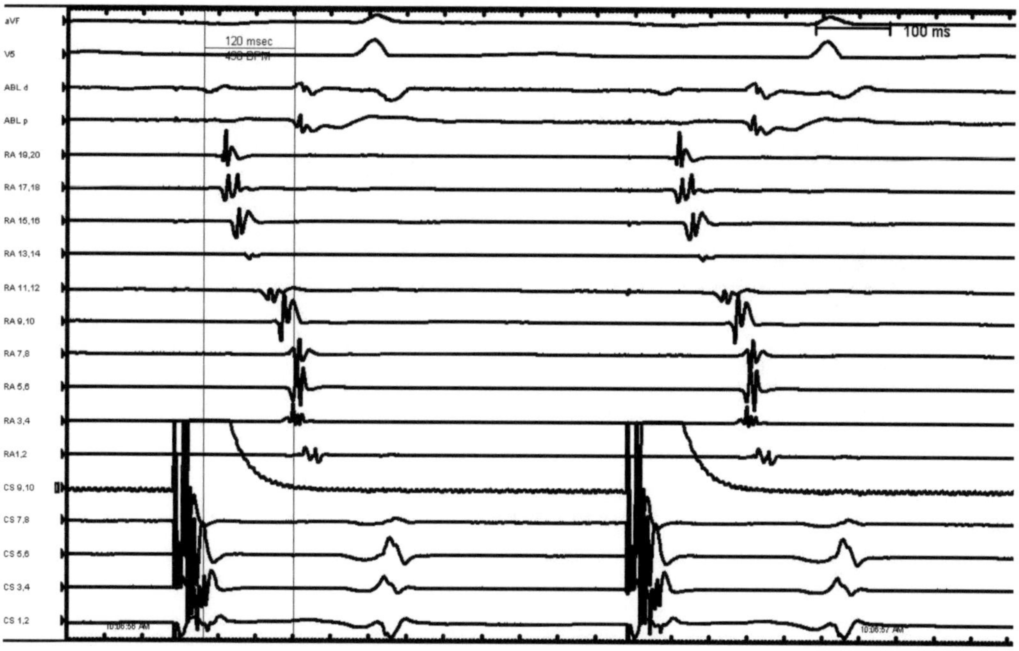

Figure 10. Online double potentials; an immediate signal post-ablation site (medial side of isthmus line) and a signal out later (lateral side of the isthmus line)

more than 50 % of the tachycardia cycle length, entrainment at multiple sites in the RA and post-pacing interval of equal or less than 30 ms including CTI and right free wall but not RA septum. Variability in LA cycle length with relatively fixed RA cycle length is also a clue that atypical flutter is localised to the right atrium.

6.7.2. Localising Atypical Flutter to the Left Atrium

Electrogram activation is usually, but not exclusively, distal to proximal on the CS catheter with passive RA conduction, or early septal RA activation, indicating breakthrough to the RA from the LA. Entrainment within the RA at multiple sites should elicit a PPI – TCL response of more than 30 ms.

6.8. 3D or non-fluoroscopic mapping

Mapping atypical flutter with a 3D mapping system (CARTO and NavX) allows direct visualisation of the re-entrant circuit [26]. When mapping the flutter, it is important to get high resolution and to cover as much as the cycle length as possible (Figure 11). Analysing up to 80–100 points increases accuracy, and covering >90 % of the circuit allows for the whole circuit to be covered. 3D mapping can be used to demonstrate the typical activation pattern. Scar can be determined by areas of signals less than 0.5 mV or inability to pace capture at 20 mA.

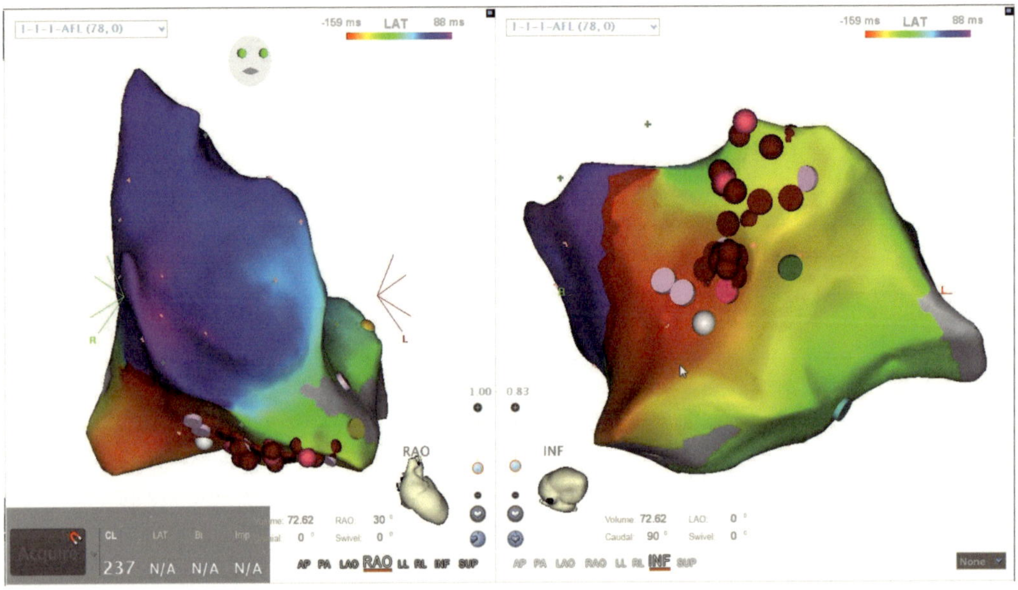

Figure 11. Figure 11: A 3-dimensional CARTO map of cavo-tricuspid isthmus-dependant atrial flutter in a patient with a history of congenital heart disease (tetralogy of Fallot, s/p repair) and symptomatic typical atrial flutter. Right anterior oblique (RAO) view and inferior view of RA demonstrating the macro-reentrant mechanism and the ablation sites

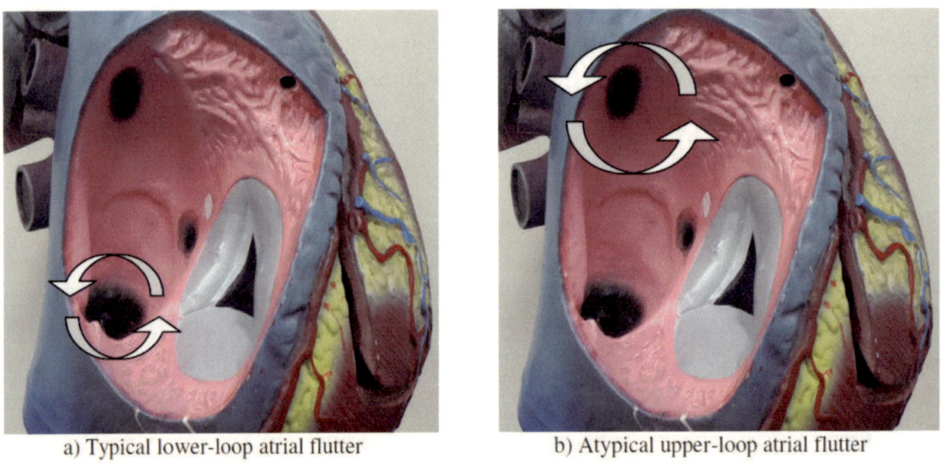

Figure 12. Activation sequence in upper-loop re-entry compared to lower-loop re-entry. Lower-loop re-entry is classified in the same group as typical atrial flutter because the circuit is dependent on CTI

6.8.1. Upper-loop re-entry atrial flutter

This atypical flutter has clockwise activation sequence around the SVC and breaks out through the crista terminalis (Figure 12). This type of flutter is typically seen in patients with hyper-

http://dx.doi.org/10.5772/60700

tension or some structural heart disease. Entrainment should be performed between the fossa ovalis and the superior vena cava (SVC) in the atrial septum. The targeted ablation site is at the excitable gap in the crista terminalis.

6.8.2. RA free wall atrial flutter

This atrial flutter is seen in patients with no structural heart disease, who develop scar in the right atria and in postsurgical patients with a scar caused by an atriotomy procedure. When mapping for the scar relating to the flutter, online double potentials will be present, and fractionation at the end of the line denotes the pivot point for the flutter. The ablative strategy for this flutter is to create a linear line from the lateral RA (at the end of the line) to the IVC or to create a line of block between the scar and the crista terminalis. It is also recommended that the cavo-tricuspid isthmus line be performed. It is important to pace in the right atrium at the proposed ablation point to avoid phrenic nerve injury.

6.8.3. LA atrial flutter

Flutter arising from the left atria is almost certainly related to the patient having some sort of structural heart disease. It is most likely to arise from the mitral annulus, the pulmonary veins or a spontaneous scar. The target ablation site for left atrial flutters depends on the circuit of the flutter and the position of the anatomical block. A new class of left atrial flutter has arisen in the recent past which is idiopathic in origin, post-pulmonary vein isolation and left atrial ablation for atrial fibrillation. This form of atrial flutter occurs between ablation lines performed to isolate and compartmentalise the left atrium to modify the burden of atrial fibrillation in patients. It has rapidly become a very common form of left atrial flutter, perhaps the most common.

7. Ablation

7.1. Radio-frequency ablation

Radio-frequency ablation uses radio-frequency energy in the form of electrical current delivered from typically 4 to 8 mm catheter tip and collects it on an indifferent electrode patch which is commonly placed on the mid-spine in the lumbar region. The density of the current at the catheter tip causes an ablation lesion 4–6 mm deep in the cardiac tissue which interrupts electrical conduction. An 8 mm catheter tip is increasingly being used as the first choice in CTI ablation due to the length and depth of ablation line needed. Irrigated catheters with a shorter tip length of 3.5–4 mm are employed in redo cases where deeper ablation lesions are needed.

In the management of especially typical atrial flutter, ablation has evolved as the first-line treatment, even after a single episode of documented symptomatic atrial flutter above antiarrhythmic pharmacotherapy [27]. In this multicentric prospective randomised study, amiodarone and radio-frequency ablation were compared in 104 patients (aged 78 +/-5 years; 20 women) with atrial flutter. The recurrence of atrial flutter was 3.8 % versus 29.5 %, P<0.0001.

Ablation therapy for atrial flutter has a success rate depending on the studies of ~90–95 % [28]. The other forms of atrial flutter generally also respond best to ablation if the circuit can be mapped and a line of conduction is performed.

The conventional method of CTI ablation was to make a linear ablation line along CTI as guided by electrograms; however recently, the 'maximum voltage-guided' technique using radio-frequency application has been studied as an alternative method and has demonstrated to be equivocal in achieving bidirectional cavo-tricuspid isthmus block. Ablation for atrial flutter using the "Maximum Voltage Guided" technique results in significantly less ablation applications than the traditional approach, potentially by concentrating ablation lesions on the muscle bundles responsible for Trans-isthmus conduction [29, 30].

7.2. Complications

During ablation, signs that can indicate that the catheter is ablating in a possibly unsafe position can include ventricular ectopy or a sharp increase in measured catheter tip impedance. Ventricular ectopy could indicate that the ablation catheter is in close proximity to the tricuspid annulus or right ventricle and potentially result in valve damage. A sharp impedance rise could indicate that the catheter has been pulled back into the IVC or wedged into a pouch on the isthmus which can create a sharp temperate increase and a possibility of a steam pop.

In patients who have had persistent atrial flutter, ablation can result in post-reversion asystole. This is commonly due to underlying sinus node disease. So one should always be ready to pace in either the atria (assuming normal AV node conduction) or ventricle (assuming a ventricular catheter is in place). Rarely, cavo-tricuspid isthmus ablation can lead to atrioventricular block or myocardial infarction if the right coronary artery or the artery to the atrioventricular node is occluded by an ablation lesion.

Other complications which can potentially occur during atrial flutter ablation include venous access/puncture (one in 100) such as hematoma, bruising and deep vein thrombosis, with or without pulmonary embolism. A small risk of stroke (1 in 500), pericardial effusion or death (1 in 1,000) remains with radio-frequency ablation method.

7.3. Emerging trends and novel technologies

Recently, the focus of atrial flutter ablation has been on emerging technology. There has been some promising data about the use of contact force catheter and its effectiveness at predicting the lesion size using the lesion size index (LSI). It is based on an algorithm which integrates contact force, radio-frequency power and ablation duration to make a key parameter, force-time integral [31]. Contact force catheters are used for pulmonary vein isolation. Contact force parameters however have not yet been employed for atrial flutter ablation. We are currently involved in a research study of a contact force catheter, and the initial results have shown that the guidance of CTI ablation using novel CF parameters can be performed successfully. It is independent of traditional parameters and demonstrates excellent short- to medium-term results.

http://dx.doi.org/10.5772/60700

8. Other ablation modalities

Cryoablation is another ablation modality which also has a good success rate with a 10 % recurrence rate [32]. The short- and long-term results are comparable to RFA, and it is relatively pain-free.

Microwave ablation has been used successfully to cure atrial fibrillation during open-heart surgery, and it has been demonstrated to be safe and effective in a preliminary feasibility study [33].

High-frequency ultrasound and diode laser balloon ablation catheter [34] have shown some promising results in the treatment of atrial fibrillation [35]. The use of these technologies in treatment of atrial flutter needs further research.

9. Conclusions

Atrial flutter is a common atrial arrhythmia with a characteristic mechanism. Its morbidity and mortality are similar to atrial fibrillation; but unlike atrial fibrillation, it can be cured. However, a thorough understanding of electrophysiological properties and anatomical landmarks is essential in achieving a successful ablation outcome and in reducing complication rates. The advent of newer technology potentially has a favourable outlook in reducing the time required to perform the procedure.

Author details

Shameer Ahmed, Andrew Claughton and Paul A. Gould*

*Address all correspondence to: drpgould@gmail.com

Department of Cardiology Princess Alexandra Hospital, University of Queensland, Brisbane, Australia

References

[1] Granada J, Uribe W, Chyou PH, Maassen K, Vierkant R, Smith PN, et al. Incidence and predictors of atrial flutter in the general population. Journal of the American College of Cardiology. 2000 Dec;36(7):2242-6. PubMed PMID: 11127467.

[2] Medi C, Kalman JM. Prediction of the atrial flutter circuit location from the surface electrocardiogram. Europace : European Pacing, Arrhythmias, and Cardiac Electrophysiology : Journal of the Working Groups on Cardiac Pacing, Arrhythmias, and

Cardiac Cellular Electrophysiology of the European Society of Cardiology. 2008 Jul; 10(7):786-96. PubMed PMID: 18456647.

[3] Wells JL, Jr., MacLean WA, James TN, Waldo AL. Characterization of atrial flutter. studies in man after open heart surgery using fixed atrial electrodes. Circulation. 1979 Sep;60(3):665-73. PubMed PMID: 455626

[4] Saoudi N, Cosio F, Waldo A, Chen SA, Iesaka Y, Lesh M, et al. A classification of atrial flutter and regular atrial tachycardia according to electrophysiological mechanisms and anatomical bases; A Statement from a Joint Expert Group from The Working Group of Arrhythmias of the European Society of Cardiology and the North American Society of Pacing and Electrophysiology. European Heart Journal. 2001 Jul;22(14):1162-82. PubMed PMID: 11440490

[5] Cosio FG, Arribas F, Lopez-Gil M, Gonzalez HD. Radiofrequency ablation of atrial flutter. Journal of Cardiovascular Electrophysiology. 1996 Jan;7(1):60-70. PubMed PMID: 8718985.

[6] Saoudi N, Nair M, Abdelazziz A, Poty H, Daou A, Anselme F, et al. Electrocardiographic patterns and results of radiofrequency catheter ablation of clockwise type I atrial flutter. Journal of Cardiovascular Electrophysiology. 1996 Oct;7(10):931-42. PubMed PMID: 8894935.

[7] SippensGroenewegen A, Lesh MD, Roithinger FX, Ellis WS, Steiner PR, Saxon LA, et al. Body surface mapping of counterclockwise and clockwise typical atrial flutter: a comparative analysis with endocardial activation sequence mapping. Journal of the American College of Cardiology. 2000 Apr;35(5):1276-87. PubMed PMID: 10758970.

[8] Zhang S, Younis G, Hariharan R, Ho J, Yang Y, Ip J, et al. Lower loop reentry as a mechanism of clockwise right atrial flutter. Circulation. 2004 Apr 6;109(13):1630-5. PubMed PMID: 15037534.

[9] Tomita Y, Matsuo K, Sahadevan J, Khrestian CM, Waldo AL. Role of functional block extension in lesion-related atrial flutter. Circulation. 2001 Feb 20;103(7):1025-30. PubMed PMID: 11181480.

[10] Cheng J, Scheinman MM. Acceleration of typical atrial flutter due to double-wave reentry induced by programmed electrical stimulation. Circulation. 1998 Apr 28;97(16): 1589-96. PubMed PMID: 9593564.

[11] Campbell M. The paroxysmal tachycardias. Lancet. 1947 Nov 1;2(6479):641; passim. PubMed PMID: 20268699.

[12] Blomstrom-Lundqvist C, Scheinman MM, Aliot EM, Alpert JS, Calkins H, Camm AJ, et al. ACC/AHA/ESC guidelines for the management of patients with supraventricular arrhythmias--executive summary. a report of the American college of cardiology/ American heart association task force on practice guidelines and the European society of cardiology committee for practice guidelines (writing committee to develop guidelines for the management of patients with supraventricular arrhythmias) devel-

oped in collaboration with NASPE-Heart Rhythm Society. Journal of the American College of Cardiology. 2003 Oct 15;42(8):1493-531. PubMed PMID: 14563598.

[13] Smit MD, Crijns HJ, Tijssen JG, Hillege HL, Alings M, Tuininga YS, et al. Effect of lenient versus strict rate control on cardiac remodeling in patients with atrial fibrillation data of the RACE II (RAte Control Efficacy in permanent atrial fibrillation II) study. Journal of the American College of Cardiology. 2011 Aug 23;58(9):942-9. PubMed PMID: 21851883.

[14] Hagens VE, Vermeulen KM, TenVergert EM, Van Veldhuisen DJ, Bosker HA, Kamp O, et al. Rate control is more cost-effective than rhythm control for patients with persistent atrial fibrillation--results from the RAte Control versus Electrical cardioversion (RACE) study. European Heart Journal. 2004 Sep;25(17):1542-9. PubMed PMID: 15342174.

[15] Singh S, Zoble RG, Yellen L, Brodsky MA, Feld GK, Berk M, et al. Efficacy and safety of oral dofetilide in converting to and maintaining sinus rhythm in patients with chronic atrial fibrillation or atrial flutter: the symptomatic atrial fibrillation investigative research on dofetilide (SAFIRE-D) study. Circulation. 2000 Nov 7;102(19): 2385-90. PubMed PMID: 11067793.

[16] Naccarelli GV, Dorian P, Hohnloser SH, Coumel P. Prospective comparison of flecainide versus quinidine for the treatment of paroxysmal atrial fibrillation/flutter. The Flecainide Multicenter Atrial Fibrillation Study Group. The American Journal of Cardiology. 1996 Jan 25;77(3):53A-9A. PubMed PMID: 8607392.

[17] You JJ, Singer DE, Howard PA, Lane DA, Eckman MH, Fang MC, et al. Antithrombotic therapy for atrial fibrillation: Antithrombotic Therapy and Prevention of Thrombosis, 9th ed: American College of Chest Physicians Evidence-Based Clinical Practice Guidelines. Chest. 2012 Feb;141(2 Suppl):e531S-75S. PubMed PMID: 22315271. Pubmed Central PMCID: 3278056.

[18] Odum LE, Cochran KA, Aistrope DS, Snella KA. The CHADS(2)versus the new CHA2DS2-VASc scoring systems for guiding antithrombotic treatment of patients with atrial fibrillation: review of the literature and recommendations for use. Pharmacotherapy. 2012 Mar;32(3):285-96. PubMed PMID: 22392459.

[19] Alyeshmerni D, Pirmohamed A, Barac A, Smirniotopoulos J, Xue E, Goldstein S, et al. Transesophageal echocardiographic screening before atrial flutter ablation: is it necessary for patient safety? Journal of the American Society of Echocardiography : Official Publication of the American Society of Echocardiography. 2013 Sep;26(9): 1099-105. PubMed PMID: 23850522.

[20] Waldo AL. Atrial flutter: entrainment characteristics. Journal of Cardiovascular Electrophysiology. 1997 Mar;8(3):337-52. PubMed PMID: 9083885.

[21] Chen J, De Chillou C, Basiouny T, Sadoul N, Filho JD, Magnin-Poull I, et al. Cavotricuspid isthmus mapping to assess bidirectional block during common atrial flutter

radiofrequency ablation. Circulation. 1999 Dec 21-28;100(25):2507-13. PubMed PMID: 10604888.

[22] Chen J, De Chillou C, Hoff PI, Rossvoll O, Andronache M, Sadoul N, et al. Identification of extremely slow conduction in the cavotricuspid isthmus during common atrial flutter ablation. Journal of Interventional Cardiac Electrophysiology : An International Journal of Arrhythmias and Pacing. 2002 Aug;7(1):67-75. PubMed PMID: 12391422.

[23] Tai CT, Haque A, Lin YK, Tsao HM, Ding YA, Chang MS, et al. Double potential interval and transisthmus conduction time for prediction of cavotricuspid isthmus block after ablation of typical atrial flutter. Journal of Interventional Cardiac Electrophysiology : An International Journal of Arrhythmias and Pacing. 2002 Aug;7(1): 77-82. PubMed PMID: 12391423.

[24] Shah D, Haissaguerre M, Takahashi A, Jais P, Hocini M, Clementy J. Differential pacing for distinguishing block from persistent conduction through an ablation line. Circulation. 2000 Sep 26;102(13):1517-22. PubMed PMID: 11004142.

[25] Cosio FG, Awamleh P, Pastor A, Nunez A. Determining inferior vena cava-tricuspid isthmus block after typical atrial flutter ablation. Heart Rhythm : The Official Journal of the Heart Rhythm Society. 2005 Mar;2(3):328-32. PubMed PMID: 15851329.

[26] Shah DC, Jais P, Haissaguerre M, Chouairi S, Takahashi A, Hocini M, et al. Three-dimensional mapping of the common atrial flutter circuit in the right atrium. Circulation. 1997 Dec 2;96(11):3904-12. PubMed PMID: 9403614.

[27] Da Costa A, Thevenin J, Roche F, Romeyer-Bouchard C, Abdellaoui L, Messier M, et al. Results from the Loire-Ardeche-Drome-Isere-Puy-de-Dome (LADIP) trial on atrial flutter, a multicentric prospective randomized study comparing amiodarone and radiofrequency ablation after the first episode of symptomatic atrial flutter. Circulation. 2006 Oct 17;114(16):1676-81. PubMed PMID: 17030680.

[28] Calkins H, Yong P, Miller JM, Olshansky B, Carlson M, Saul JP, et al. Catheter ablation of accessory pathways, atrioventricular nodal reentrant tachycardia, and the atrioventricular junction: final results of a prospective, multicenter clinical trial. The Atakr Multicenter Investigators Group. Circulation. 1999 Jan 19;99(2):262-70. PubMed PMID: 9892593.

[29] Gula LJ, Redfearn DP, Veenhuyzen GD, Krahn AD, Yee R, Klein GJ, et al. Reduction in atrial flutter ablation time by targeting maximum voltage: results of a prospective randomized clinical trial. Journal of Cardiovascular Electrophysiology. 2009 Oct; 20(10):1108-12. PubMed PMID: 19549033.

[30] Sato H, Yagi T, Namekawa A, Ishida A, Yamashina Y, Nakagawa T, et al. Efficacy of bundle ablation for cavotricuspid isthmus-dependent atrial flutter: combination of the maximum voltage-guided ablation technique and high-density electro-anatomi-

http://dx.doi.org/10.5772/60700

cal mapping. Journal of Interventional Cardiac Electrophysiology : An International Journal of Arrhythmias and Pacing. 2010 Jun;28(1):39-44. PubMed PMID: 20177759.

[31] Squara F, Latcu DG, Massaad Y, Mahjoub M, Bun SS, Saoudi N. Contact force and force-time integral in atrial radiofrequency ablation predict transmurality of lesions. Europace : European Pacing, Arrhythmias, and Cardiac Electrophysiology : Journal of the Working Groups on Cardiac Pacing, Arrhythmias, and Cardiac Cellular Electrophysiology of the European Society of Cardiology. 2014 May;16(5):660-7. PubMed PMID: 24798957.

[32] Manusama R, Timmermans C, Limon F, Philippens S, Crijns HJ, Rodriguez LM. Catheter-based cryoablation permanently cures patients with common atrial flutter. Circulation. 2004 Apr 6;109(13):1636-9. PubMed PMID: 15023886.

[33] Chan JY, Fung JW, Yu CM, Feld GK. Preliminary results with percutaneous transcatheter microwave ablation of typical atrial flutter. Journal of Cardiovascular Electrophysiology. 2007 Mar;18(3):286-9. PubMed PMID: 17284286.

[34] Reddy VY, Houghtaling C, Fallon J, Fischer G, Farr N, Clarke J, et al. Use of a diode laser balloon ablation catheter to generate circumferential pulmonary venous lesions in an open-thoracotomy caprine model. Pacing and Clinical Electrophysiology : PACE. 2004 Jan;27(1):52-7. PubMed PMID: 14720155.

[35] Burkhardt JD, Natale A. New technologies in atrial fibrillation ablation. Circulation. 2009 Oct 13;120(15):1533-41. PubMed PMID: 19822816.

Chapter 2

Recent Advances in the Noninvasive Study of Atrial Conduction Defects Preceding Atrial Fibrillation

Raúl Alcaraz and José Joaquín Rieta

Additional information is available at the end of the chapter

http://dx.doi.org/10.5772/60729

Abstract

The P-wave represents the electrical activity in the electrocardiogram (ECG) associated with the heart's atrial contraction. This wave has merited significant research efforts in recent years with the aim to characterize atrial depolarization from the ECG. Indeed, the alterations of the P-wave main time, frequency, and wavelet features have been widely studied to predict the onset of atrial fibrillation (AF), both spontaneously and after a specific treatment, such as pharmacological or electrical cardioversion, catheter ablation, as well as cardiac surgery. To this respect, the P-wave prolongation is today a clinically accepted marker of high risk of suffering AF. However, given the relatively low P-wave amplitude in the ECG, its analysis has been most widely carried out from signal-averaged ECG signals. Unfortunately, these kind of recordings are uncommon in routine clinical practice and, moreover, they obstruct the possibility of studying the information carried by each single P-wave as well as its variability over time. These limitations have motivated the recent development of the beat-to-beat P-wave analysis, which has proven to be very useful in revealing interesting information about the altered atrial conduction preceding the onset of AF. Within this context, the main goal of this chapter is to review the most recent advances reached by this kind of analysis in the noninvasive assessment of atrial conduction alterations. Thus, the chapter will introduce and discuss the existing methods of the beat-to-beat P-wave analysis and their application to predict the onset of AF as well as its advantages and disadvantages compared with the signal-averaged P-wave analysis.

Keywords: atrial premature contractions, electrocardiogram, paroxysmal atrial fibrillation, P-wave, variability

1. Introduction

Atrial fibrillation (AF) has been described as the arrhythmia of the twenty-first century given that it is the most commonly diagnosed sustained cardiac arrhythmia, affecting up to 1% of the general population and up to 15% of the population older than 70 years of age [1, 2]. Despite extensive research during the last decades, it is still unclear how AF starts and perpetuates itself [2]. Once AF appears, its usual evolution presents three different stages [3]. In the first one, named paroxysmal AF (PAF), patients present auto-limited episodes with a duration shorter than seven days, which terminate spontaneously without the need of medical intervention. However, approximately between 15 and 31% of PAF patients progress to permanent AF in four to eight years [4]. During this progression, recurrent episodes normally appear, but it is also still unknown why the duration of these episodes varies from patient to patient and from episode to episode [5]. Therefore, once a PAF episode has terminated spontaneously, the early prediction of the onset of the next PAF episode is a relevant clinical challenge. Such a prediction may minimize risks for AF patients and improve their quality of life, since a preventive therapy may be used to avoid recurrence of the arrhythmia. Thus, the maintenance of normal sinus rhythm may reduce symptoms, get better hemodynamics, and minimize the atrial remodeling, which increases the probability of recurrence of AF [6]. Moreover, the risk of suffering thromboembolic events can also be notably reduced [2].

The normal electrical conduction in the heart is generated by the sinoatrial node and is propagated throughout the right atrium and through the Bachmann's bundle to the left atrium, thus defining the P-wave in the electrocardiogram (ECG). However, when this progressive conduction is altered by accessory pathways, reentries, or conduction delays, the P-wave morphology will reflect this fact [7]. Currently, it is well known that both slowed conduction velocity as well as inhomogeneous cell refractory periods in several atrial regions are atrial electrophysiological alterations provoking and maintaining AF [8]. Such atrial conduction abnormalities result in prolonged and highly variable P-waves [9]. Thereby, the analysis of the P-wave has gained increasing interest in the last years [10].

Within this context, the noninvasive P-wave analysis has been performed, following two main recording approaches. On the one hand, it has been based on the standard 12-lead ECG [11]. On the other hand, some authors have based their studies on the P-wave vector magnitude obtained from Frank's orthogonal leads [12]. However, in both alternatives, only averaged-signal P-waves have been widely analyzed in order to minimize the shortcomings derived from the relatively low amplitude of this wave in the ECG [13]. Indeed, the duration of the averaged P-wave has been widely analyzed, and its prolongation has been associated with history of AF, development of arrhythmia after bypass surgery, and progression from paroxysmal to persistent AF [9]. Additionally, the fragmentation of the P-wave template has also been broadly studied from the spectral, gaussian, and wavelet domains [14, 15, 16]. In this case, a wide variety of features associated with the P-wave morphology have provided the ability to discern between PAF patients and healthy subjects [15, 16], to quantify the effects of different antiarrhythmic drugs [17], and to stratify the risk of recurrence of AF after electrical cardioversion [14], catheter ablation [18, 19], and coronary artery bypass grafting [20].

However, recording of the signal-averaged P-wave is not today a common practice in the clinical routine [21]. Moreover, this kind of analysis does not allow to exploit the information contained in every individual P-wave. Indeed, consecutive P-wave averaging hinders the interesting possibility of characterizing every single P-wave as well as its variability across time. Furthermore, the ability of all the previously defined signal-averaged P-wave features to stratify the risk of PAF has also proven to be seriously reduced when long-term ECG recordings, longer than 30 minutes, with no more than two or three available leads are analyzed [22, 23, 24]. Hence, further studies are required to tackle the crucial issue about the minimum time gap required between the detection of P-wave feature alterations that potentially would provoke the onset of PAF. Within this context, recent works have introduced new alternatives able to assess the P-wave time and spatial variability from routine clinical recordings. Some of these methods have proven to accurately anticipate the risk of arrhythmia, at least 60 minutes before its onset, which is a relevant advance in turning clinically useful PAF risk predictors [25, 26, 27]. Overall, the purpose of this chapter is to describe the most recent advances presented in the literature for the noninvasive assessment of atrial conduction defects and how the information provided by these methods has allowed significant advances in the prediction of PAF onset from the surface ECG.

2. Analysis of atrial premature complexes

Several studies have shown that most PAF episodes are initiated by the presence of rapidly firing atrial ectopic foci [28, 29]. Given that their occurrence results in premature atrial depolarizations [30], the identification of a wide number of premature atrial complexes (PACs) in the ECG has proved to be a successful predictor of imminent PAF onset [31, 32]. To this respect, Thong et al. [31] defined an isolated PAC as those preceded and followed by two cycles of the prevalent rhythm. Moreover, they identified four separate categories of isolated PACs. First, Fig. 1(a) shows a PAC with sinus node reset. The sinus node is reset by the ectopic P-wave within normal conduction time, thus provoking that the next RR interval is within 100 ms of the prevalent one. Second, Fig. 1(b) shows an interpolated PAC. In this case, the sinus node is not reset and the corresponding QRS is located in a normal RR interval with no alteration of the prevalent rhythm. Third, Fig. 1(c) shows a PAC in which the sinus node reset has been delayed. A delay occurs in the path of electrical conduction to the sinus node, thus increasing the next RR interval by approximately 100 ms. Finally, Fig. 1(d) displays a PAC in which a full compensatory pause occurs. In this case, the PAC causes the AV junction to be refractory, thus doubling the RR interval compared with the prevalent one.

Making use of the database proposed by the Computers in Cardiology Challenge, which is freely available in PhysioNet [33], the authors compared the two provided ECG leads to detect rhythm changes. These rhythm changes were associated with the ECG intervals preceding the immediate onset of PAF, while those intervals more than 45 minutes far from a PAF episode were related to a normal rhythm. The authors counted the number of isolated PACs in categories 2–4 for each lead of every subject and followed the criteria presented in Fig. 2 to identify rhythm changes. Three or more consecutive PACs without any intervening long

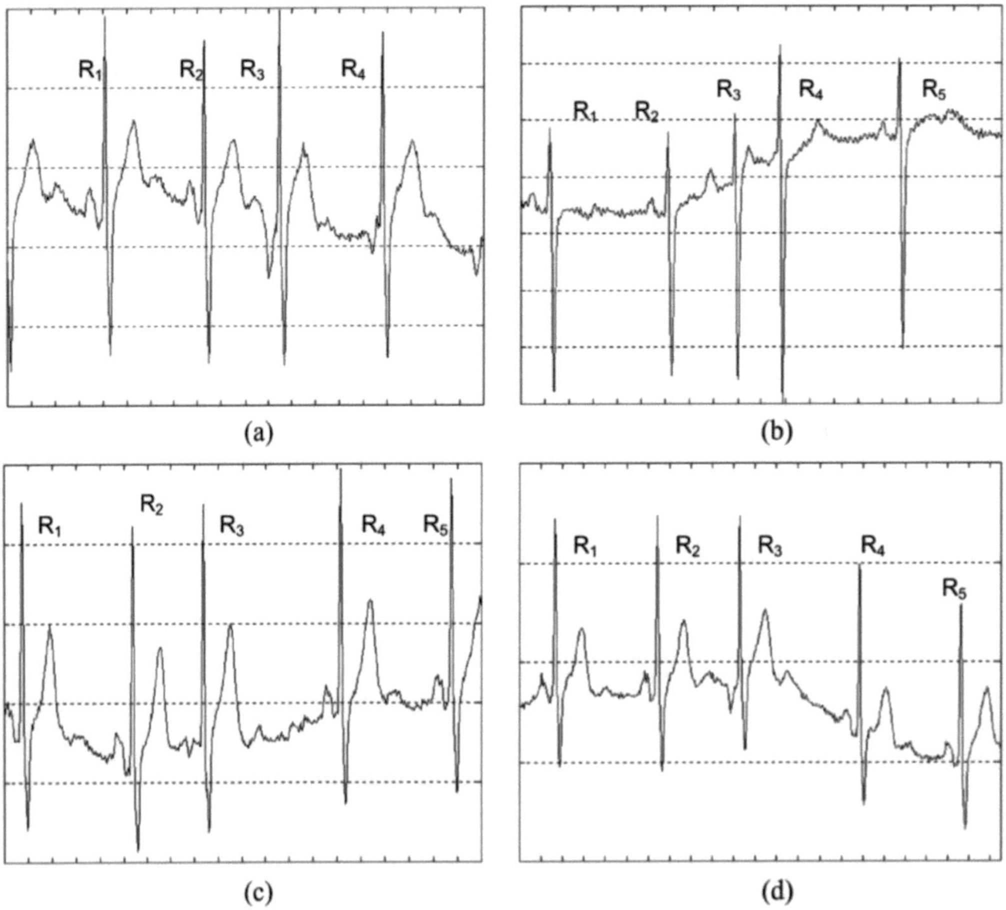

Figure 1. ECGs of various types of PACs according to Thong et al. [31]. (a) PAC with sinus reset, $R_3R_4=R_1R_2$. (b) Interpolated PAC, $R_2R_4=R_1R_2$. (c) PAC with delayed sinus node reset, $R_3R_4>R_1R_2$. (d) PAC with full compensatory pause, $R_2R_4=2R_1R_2$. QRS of PACs are similar to other QRS. RR timing is used to differentiate the four types of PACs. Note inverted P-waves in (a), (c), and (d). Horizontal tick marks are 200 ms apart.

intervals were considered to meet the PAT criterion. Regarding the PAC test, if the difference in the number of PACs between the two leads of a subject was higher than or equal to two, a rhythm change was marked. Finally, to account for atrial bigeminies and trigeminies, changes in RR series higher than 70 ms were first detected. After, a 10-point boxcar filter was applied to the RR series and the averaged power of the filtered signal was computed. A change of rhythm was detected when the average power was higher than 0.95 and a difference between leads was higher than 1.5. Finally, the algorithm allowed to discern between ECG intervals far from PAF and close to PAF with an accuracy around 90%.

This result was greater than those achieved by other participants in the Computers in Cardiology Challenge, which proposed different algorithms to detect the presence of PACs. Thus,

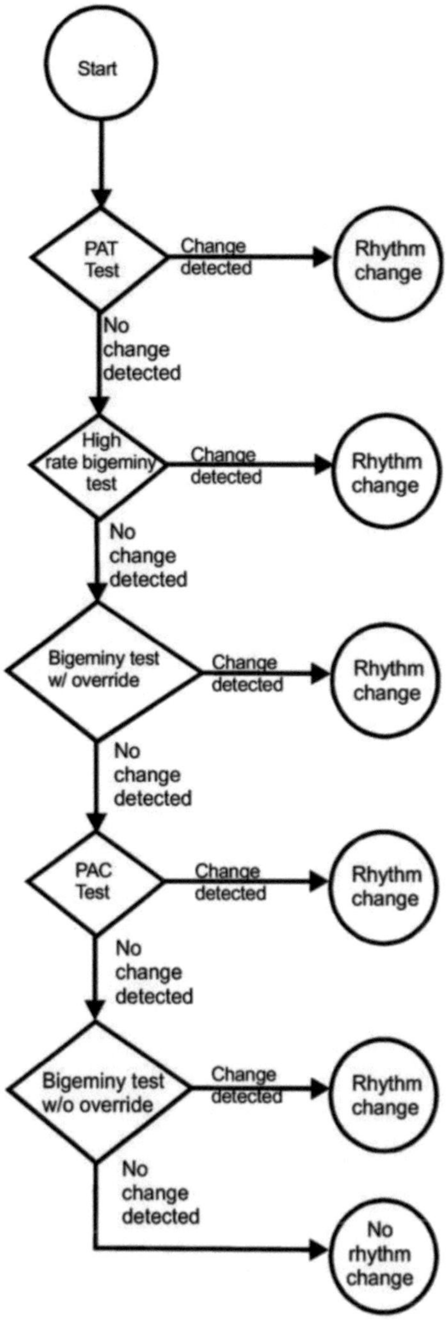

Figure 2. Flow diagram for the algorithm proposed by Thong et al. [31] to identify the onset of PAF.

Langley et al. [34] identified the potential ectopics from those provoking RR intervals shorter than 80% of their average. Next, those beats with an RR value exceeding ±10% of their mean were considered as atrial, whereas those altering more than ±30% of that value were considered as ventricular. In [35], a morphological comparison among potential ectopic and normal beat was also considered. Finally, ectopic beats were considered as those with a QRS morphology similar to normal beats. In a similar line, Schreier et al. [36] considered that those beats with a very different morphology compared to their neighbors could cause the onset of PAF. On the other hand, symbolic analysis was applied to the RR series to identify acceleration and decelerations in the heart rate and associate them with the onset of PAF. Finally, Hickey et al. [32] identified APCs by using an algorithm based on two steps. First, a beat was flagged as a suspected APC if the RR interval preceding it was 15% shorter than a defined local moving average of the surrounding RR intervals. In the second stage, the area, width, and amplitude of the QRS were computed. If all these parameters differed more than 10% from a normal beat, they were confirmed as APCs. The first 100 beats from a regular sinus rhythm were used to compute the parameters associated with normal beats. This algorithm is based on the fact that ventricular ectopics present morphologies very different from normal beats. Although the accuracy of this algorithm to identify ECG intervals immediately before the onset of PAF was slightly lower than those presented by Thong et al.'s algorithm, its combination with information obtained from the RR series spectral analysis yielded a better outcome (i.e., an accuracy around 98%) [32]. Indeed, subjects with imminent PAF showed to have highly correlated low-frequency and high-frequency components in their heart rate. Thus, the authors suggested that sympathetic and parasympathetic autonomic activity may be coupled in these subjects [32].

3. Time course of the P-wave variability

3.1. Time characterization of the P-wave

The variability of features from the P-wave time course before the onset of PAF has started to be studied very recently through a new alternative able to assess time diversity of the P-wave features from single-lead ECG recordings [25]. The method has demonstrated that the P-wave features presented an increasing variability as PAF onset approximates, thus suggesting intermittently disturbed conduction in the atrial tissue. Indeed, it is able to assess the risk of arrhythmia one hour before its onset, thus being a significant advance in the early prediction of the risk of PAF with clinical usefulness [25].

The method can be decomposed in various steps. Firstly, because no standard definition of the P-wave fiducial points can be found in the literature, the P-wave onset and offset were determined by an automatic delineator [37]. It is important to note that the delineator had the ability to deal also with ectopic beats in the same way as with normal beats [37]. Therefore, P-wave fiducial points that originated from APCs were automatically detected without any additional requirement.

After its delineation, several P-wave time features were defined as potential indicators that might be of interest for PAF onset prognosis in a beat-to-beat way, as shown in Fig. 3. To this respect, the P-wave duration was defined as the distance between its offset and onset, i.e.,

$$P_{dur} = P_{off} - P_{on}. \tag{1}$$

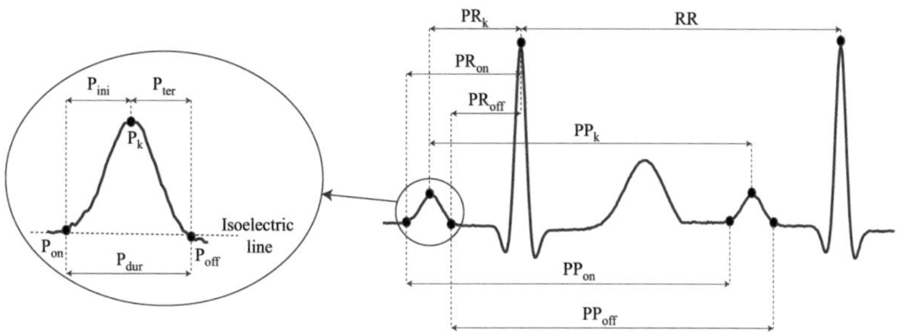

Figure 3. Visual description of the chosen parameters to characterize P-wave time features and assess its time course variation.

Previous works have demonstrated that increased P-wave duration can be considered as an indicator of increased risk of AF [11, 38, 39, 40]. In a similar way, the P-wave morphology measured from lead V1 has also shown ability to stratify the AF risk [41]. Hence, the duration of the P-wave initial and terminal portions was considered as the distances between its peak and the P-wave onset (P_{ini}) and offset (P_{ter}), respectively. Therefore, these features were defined as

$$P_{ini} = P_k - P_{on}, \tag{2}$$

and

$$P_{ter} = P_{off} - P_k. \tag{3}$$

Moreover, the P-wave asymmetry was estimated by computing the ratio between the duration of its initial and terminal portions [42], i.e.,

$$P_{asy} = \frac{P_{ter}}{P_{ini}}. \tag{4}$$

On the other hand, conduction time from the sinus node to the ventricles defines the PR interval. Thus, this interval contains information about different specific places of the atria [43]. In fact, prolongation of the PR interval has been associated with increased risk of AF in the Framingham Heart Study [43, 44]. This fact motivated the measurement of this interval from three different ways, considering the time from the onset, the peak, and the offset of the P-wave up to the R peak. This can be mathematically defined as

$$PR_{on} = R - P_{on},\tag{5}$$

$$PR_{k} = R - P_{k},\tag{6}$$

$$PR_{off} = R - P_{off}.\tag{7}$$

Finally, differences between successive P-waves were considered to estimate the P-wave location variability. In this case, three data series were also calculated. Thus, the distances among onset, peak, and offset from the i th and $i+1$ th waves were computed as

$$PP_{on} = P_{on}^{(i+1)} - P_{on}^{(i)},\tag{8}$$

$$PP_{k} = P_{k}^{(i+1)} - P_{k}^{(i)},\tag{9}$$

$$PP_{off} = P_{off}^{(i+1)} - P_{off}^{(i)}.\tag{10}$$

Once all the P-wave time features were defined, they were applied on a database of 24 patients with 24-h Holter ECG recordings. The 120 minutes preceding the onset of PAF from the longest sinus rhythm interval of every patient were extracted and divided into two 60-minute-length intervals. Moreover, a third set of 28 healthy individuals without statistically significant differences in terms of age and gender compared to the PAF patients was also analyzed. Subjects in this control group did not present any previous history of AF or structural heart disease. From each individual, a one-hour-length segment was randomly chosen.

Given the relatively low amplitude of the P-wave in the ECG, to minimize the impulsive noise in results, 10 sample-length blocks from data series for each P-wave metric were considered [25]. In each block, the variability was obtained as the difference between the 90- and 10-quantiles. On the other hand, the electrophysiological alterations occurring in the atria prior to the onset of PAF [39] provoke a great deal of scatter in the variability of the aforementioned P-wave features. To this respect, P_{dur} variability over time for a healthy subject and intervals far from PAF and close to PAF from a diseased patient are shown in Fig. 4. Then, to reduce the effect of this variability, the expected P-wave feature trend was estimated by means of a linear fitting also shown in Fig. 4. Obviously, the slope α of this fitting line provides information about the P-wave variability over time. Whereas positive α values indicate an increasing variability, a lower dispersion in the data can be indicative of negative values. Finally, α values near zero could be indicative of very reduced variability in the P-wave over time.

http://dx.doi.org/10.5772/60729

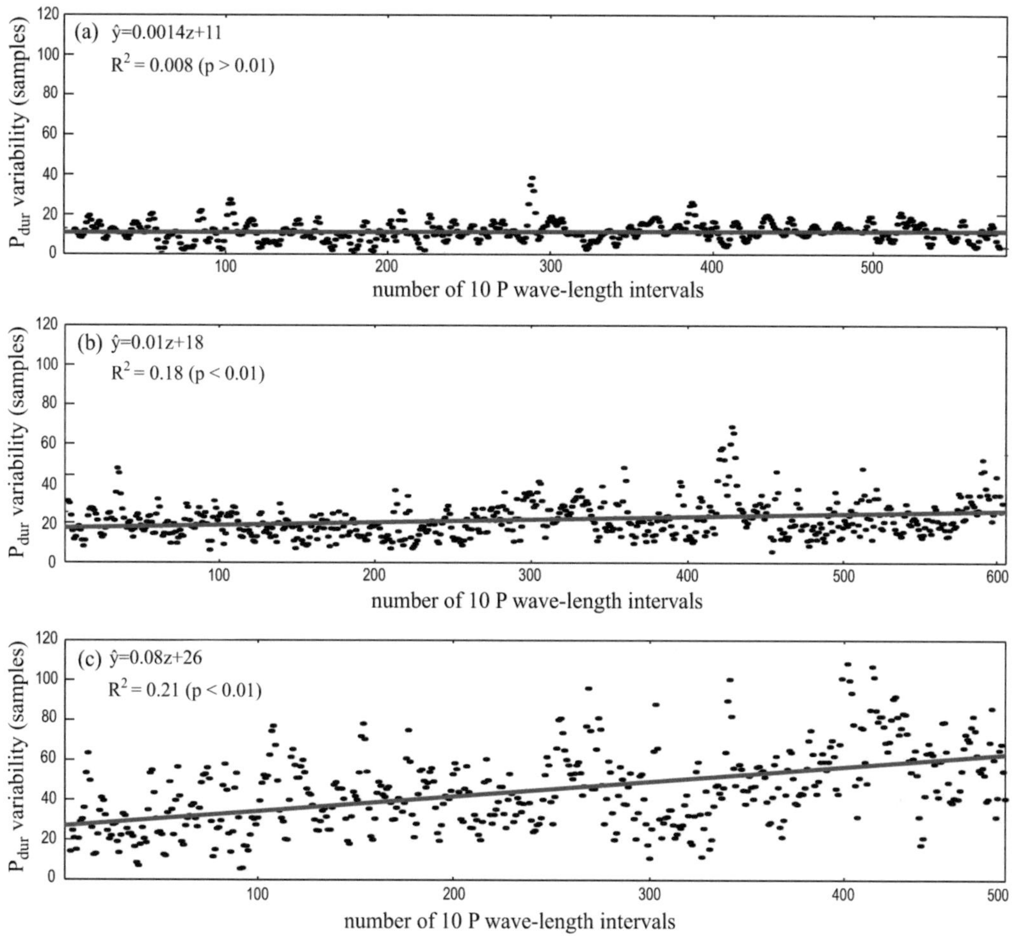

Figure 4. Typical P-wave duration variability over time from (a) a healthy individual and from ECG intervals (b) close to PAF and (c) far from PAF for a diseased patient.

Receiver operating characteristic (ROC) curves were used to obtain discriminative thresholds between the patient groups. For each P-wave feature, optimal thresholds were selected as those values of α minimizing the classification error. In the end, a stepwise discriminant analysis (SDA) was performed with the objective of improving the patient group classification.

Interestingly, for all the studied metrics, significant differences among sets were noticed, although the features measuring P-wave duration showed the most remarkable trends. Regarding the classification performance, apart from P_{ter}, metrics associated with the P-wave duration reported a higher predictive ability than the other single parameters (see Table 1). Indeed, 84.21% of all the analyzed patients were correctly identified by P_{dur}, providing among healthy subjects and PAF patients and among ECG intervals far from PAF and close to PAF accuracy values of 90.79% and 83.33%, respectively (see Fig. 5). The metric estimating the PP rhythm constituted a second set of predictive power. A global accuracy around 70% was

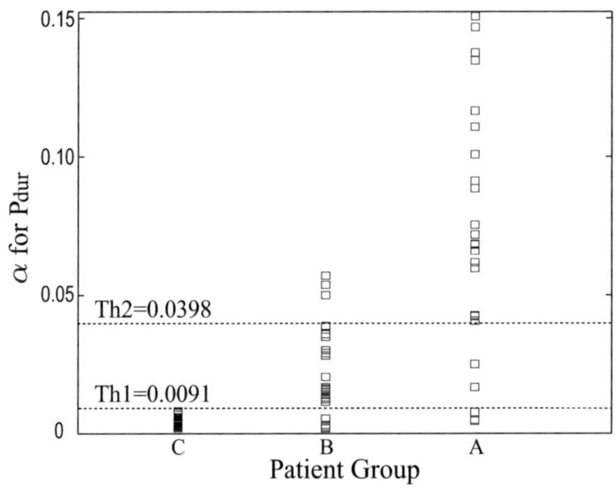

Figure 5. Classification into healthy subjects (group C), patients far from PAF (group B), and patients close to PAF (group A) making use of the P-wave duration time course.

provided by all of them, with more than 65% of the cross-validated grouped cases appropriately classified. Moreover, the RR series variability showed a classification performance very similar to PP_k and also it provided almost identical statistical differences among patients. In fact, for the three studied groups, correlation between these metrics was 0.98, 0.92, and 0.84, respectively. Finally, the most reduced ability to identify patient groups was provided by the metrics associated with the PR interval. Nevertheless, PR_{on} provided an accuracy close to the metrics computed from the PP series.

Feature	Healthy Subjects	ECGs far from PAF	ECGs close to PAF	GAcc	CV
P_{dur}	100.0% (28/28)	70.83% (17/24)	79.17% (19/24)	84.21% (64/76)	82.89% (63/76)
P_{ini}	67.86% (19/28)	70.83% (17/24)	79.17% (19/24)	72.37% (55/76)	72.37% (55/76)
P_{ter}	89.29% (25/28)	16.67% (4/24)	83.33% (20/24)	64.47% (49/76)	61.84% (47/76)
P_{asy}	96.43% (27/28)	66.67% (16/24)	75.00% (18/24)	80.26% (61/76)	78.94% (60/76)
PR_k	89.29% (25/28)	45.83% (11/24)	50.00% (12/24)	63.16% (48/76)	60.53% (46/76)
PR_{on}	85.71% (24/28)	58.33% (14/24)	62.50% (15/24)	69.74% (53/76)	68.42% (52/76)
PR_{off}	78.57% (22/28)	37.50% (9/24)	58.33% (14/24)	59.21% (45/76)	60.53% (46/76)
PP_k	82.14% (23/28)	58.33% (14/24)	70.83% (17/24)	71.05% (54/76)	69.74% (53/76)
PP_{on}	82.14% (23/28)	45.83% (11/24)	75.00% (18/24)	68.42% (52/76)	67.11% (51/76)
PP_{off}	89.29% (25/28)	33.33% (8/24)	87.50% (21/24)	71.05% (54/76)	69.74% (53/76)
RR	82.14% (23/28)	45.83% (11/24)	70.83% (17/24)	67.11% (51/76)	65.79% (50/76)
SDA (P_{dur}, PP_k)	100.0% (28/28)	83.33% (20/24)	91.67% (22/24)	92.10% (70/76)	90.79% (69/76)

Table 1. Percentage of ECG segments correctly classified for each group from the slope α obtained for each studied time P-wave feature. The table also shows the global accuracy (GAcc) and cross-validation (CV) results.

http://dx.doi.org/10.5772/60729

On the other hand, the SDA revealed an improved classification among patients from a discriminant model constructed by the combination of P_{dur} and PP_k. To this respect, as can be seen in Table 1 and Fig. 6, 92.10% of the analyzed patients were properly classified, 90.79% of cross-validated grouped cases being correctly discerned. Therefore, an increase of around 8% in the accuracy was reached in comparison with P_{dur}. Moreover, this model was also able to discern 96.05% of healthy subjects from patients suffering from PAF with a false-positive rate lower than 4%, such as can be observed in Fig. 6.

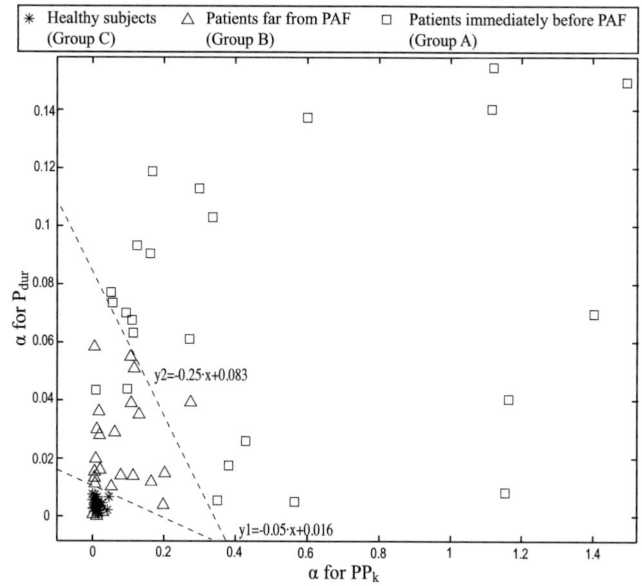

Figure 6. Classification into healthy subjects, patients far from PAF, and patients close to PAF making use of the discriminant model based on the parameters P_{dur} and PP_k. Each dotted line represents optimal discrimination thresholds between groups.

These outcomes agree with previous findings showing that prolongation of the P-wave duration is associated with history of AF [15, 38, 45, 46, 47]. Moreover, it is also worth noting that a relevant correlation between P-wave duration variability and the longest duration of the right atrial activation registered on electrograms has been previously documented [48]. Nonetheless, both for discerning among healthy subjects and PAF patients [49] and among ECG segments far from PAF and close to PAF, the beat-to-beat P-wave variability analysis over time has revealed higher discriminant ability than previous works.

The P-wave duration reflected on the ECG can be considered as the overlapped result of two effects [42]: (i) its prolongation due to the decrease in atrial conduction velocity and (ii) its shortening due to overlapping between atrial depolarization and possible premature atrial repolarization, as a result of decreased refractory period. Given that the patients prone to AF manifest a heterogeneous combination of both effects [42, 2], the observed higher P-wave duration variability preceding the onset of PAF can be considered as a natural consequence feasible to be expected. A similar behavior could also be expected for the PR interval variability over time, because that variability could reflect alterations in atrial depolarization and delays in atrioventricular node conduction. Anyway, although both parameters showed the same behavior, it has to be remarked that the P-wave duration variability was a better predictive marker. Moreover, any of the three estimates of the PR interval reported a classification higher than 70%. Nonetheless, statistically significant differences among groups were revealed by the three metrics, thus agreeing with previous works which have addressed the susceptibility to spontaneous AF [50] and post-coronary bypass surgery AF [51].

On the other hand, the notable correlation between the series of RR and PP merits special attention. This result suggests that similar information is provided by both series. However, in comparison with healthy subjects, the correlation for PAF patients was lower, thus suggesting that some information differences are revealed in this case. These differences between PP and RR series may be related to the P-wave variability before the onset of PAF, such as the aforementioned. As a consequence, the assessment of the PP series instead of the RR series is recommended to estimate the risk of PAF onset.

In recent years, a wide variety of previous works have analyzed the RR series preceding the onset of PAF to predict this event [52, 32, 53, 54, 55, 56, 57]. Whereas typical time and frequency measurements on the RR time series provided not to be relevant markers of the onset of PAF, the identification of a decreased heart rate complexity has proven ability to identify that event [52, 53, 54]. Entropy metrics such as approximate entropy and sample entropy have been mainly used to analyze RR complexity. However, the result provided by these metrics is in contrast with the previously presented increasing trend in the PP series variability. This contradictory outcomes could be justified by an incorrect use of the entropy metrics. In previous works, a notable effect of spikes on entropy metrics has been reported [58], and the increasing presence of APCs before the onset of PAF is a notable source of spikes in RR series [53]. Anyway, additional studies are required to validate this hypothesis.

On the other hand, although many studies quantifying RR complexity have presented a higher ability to predict the onset of PAF than the metrics based on PP series, they had to combine a wide variety of different indices by using very complex classifiers. To this respect, artificial neural networks, self-organization maps, support vector machines, or linear discriminant classifiers have been introduced in different studies [32, 55, 56, 57]. Obviously this kind of metrics combination hinders the direct and clinical interpretation of the results, thus obstructing the possibility to be used in daily clinical routine. On the contrary, the beat-to-beat P-wave variability analysis has revealed a simple discriminant model based on the combination of two clearly interpretable metrics such as P_{dur} and PP_k [25]. Indeed, the discriminant model suggests that the presence of a high P-wave duration and rhythm variability over time is indicative of a high risk of the onset of PAF.

3.2. Morphological characterization of the P-wave

Factors such as right and left atrial depolarization as well as the shape and size of atrial chambers determine the P-wave morphology [9]. Therefore, alterations in the P-wave morphology can be indicative of a disrupting atrial conduction [11]. Within this context, recent works have focused on quantifying the P-wave morphological variability during the two hours preceding the onset of PAF [26]. In this case, a wider database composed of 48 Holter recordings from PAF patients and 53 healthy individuals, age and gender matched, has been considered [26]. As in [25], the longest sinus rhythm interval in the recording from each patient was selected and the two-hour segment preceding the onset of PAF was analyzed. The interval under study was divided into two one-hour-length segments. Additionally, an ECG segment of one hour in length was randomly chosen from the Holter recording of each healthy subject.

In order to define the morphological features able to characterize the P-waves, it has to be considered that previous works have suggested that inhomogeneous intra-atrial and interatrial electrical conduction predisposes to the development of AF [42, 16]; therefore, maximum and minimum conduction velocities during the atrial depolarization were estimated as [42]

$$v_{\max} = \max_{n=2,3,\ldots,L} \left(\tilde{w}[n] - \tilde{w}[n-1]\right) \qquad \text{and} \tag{11}$$

$$v_{\min} = \min_{n=2,3,\ldots,L} \left(\tilde{w}[n] - \tilde{w}[n-1]\right), \tag{12}$$

respectively, $\tilde{w}[n]$ being each individual sample of the P-wave. Moreover, the dispersion in the propagation velocity during the depolarization process was also obtained as

$$v_{\text{disp}} = v_{\max} - v_{\min}. \tag{13}$$

On the other hand, altered and fractionated atrial activity seems to be reflected as the appearance of bumps in the P-wave normal gaussian shape [15], which could provoke even phase changes in lead V1 [41]. This morphology change was computed by means of the arc length of each P-wave (P_{al}), i.e.,

$$P_{al} = \sum_{n=2}^{L} \sqrt{1 + \left(\tilde{w}[n] - \tilde{w}[n-1]\right)^2}. \tag{14}$$

This metric is able to discern between two waves with the same duration but different morphologies (see Fig. 7), because it computes the rectified P-wave length. In fact, in this figure, a notably longer arc length can be observed for the wave with abnormal morphology than for those with a normal waveform.

On the other hand, the P-wave amplitude has been widely analyzed in previous works. Indeed, various authors have suggested a relationship between this metric and the electrical mass depolarized in each atrial beat, thus showing a significant decrease after pulmonary vein ablation [59] and external electrical cardioversion [14]. Overall, several metrics to quantify this

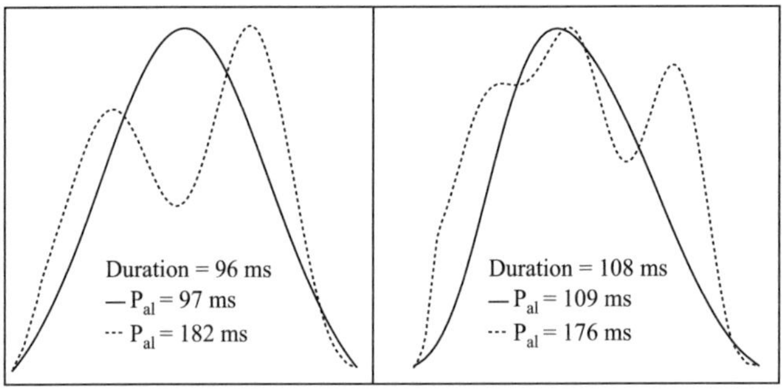

Figure 7. Representative P-waves showing different morphologies but similar lengths. As can be observed, the P-wave arc length is able to discern between the two different morphologies.

amplitude have been proposed in the literature [26]. To this respect, two robust parameters are based on computing the normalized root mean square value and the area of the P-wave as

$$P_{nrms} = \sqrt{\frac{1}{L}\sum_{n=1}^{L}\tilde{w}[n]^2} \quad \text{and} \tag{15}$$

$$P_{area} = \sum_{n=1}^{L}\left|\tilde{w}[n]\right|, \tag{16}$$

respectively. Finally, to avoid the effect of the P-wave duration on its amplitude, both parameters have been also normalized as follows:

$$P_{nenergy} = \frac{P_{nrms}^{\ 2}}{P_{al}}, \quad P_{narea} = \frac{P_{area}}{P_{al}} \tag{17}$$

The variability of these parameters over the one-hour-length recordings was estimated in the same way as in the previous subsection. However, the performance of each single-parameter variability to discriminate between ECG segments far from and close to PAF and healthy subjects was evaluated by means of a stratified 2-fold cross-validation. The results are summarized in Table 2. In this case, more than 82% of the healthy subjects were identified by all the metrics. Additionally, P_{al} and P_{area} discerned between ECG intervals far from PAF and close to PAF with a accuracy greater than 60% and 70%, respectively. Thus, the greatest global accuracy around 80% was reached by the P-wave arc length, also presenting accuracy values of 94.48% and 86.96% among healthy individuals and PAF patients and among ECG intervals far from PAF and close to PAF, respectively. The second highest discriminant ability was presented by the P-wave area, which reported a global accuracy slightly higher than 75% in the test sets.

Feature	Healthy subjects		Far from PAF		Close to PAF		Global Accuracy	
	training	test	training	test	training	test	training	test
v_{max}	90.01%	86.95%	55.22%	42.17%	57.83%	52.61%	68.76%	61.86%
v_{min}	90.58%	87.96%	45.00%	35.87%	63.48%	56.52%	67.52%	61.46%
v_{disp}	90.60%	88.60%	40.22%	35.87%	73.91%	71.74%	69.30%	66.55%
P_{al}	96.62%	89.98%	79.57%	68.75%	84.78%	79.79%	87.45%	80.02%
P_{nrms}	86.82%	83.82%	58.26%	52.39%	69.35%	65.87%	72.22%	68.15%
P_{area}	90.72%	87.76%	70.22%	60.91%	75.22%	70.87%	79.31%	75.24%
$P_{nenergy}$	86.42%	82.94%	51.52%	40.65%	73.04%	62.83%	71.10%	63.16%
P_{narea}	89.05%	86.58%	55.43%	46.09%	72.83%	67.17%	73.23%	67.58%

Table 2. Percentage of ECG segments correctly classified for each group from the slope α obtained for each studied morphological P-wave feature.

Moreover, a decision tree was assembled to investigate non-monotonic relationships among single parameters, thus improving group classification. This tree showed that the optimal combination of parameters was also achieved by the P-wave arc length and area. Figure 8 shows the obtained decision tree. As can be observed, low P-wave area variability identified healthy individuals. On the contrary, increasing variability in P-wave area and arc length over time was observed when the onset of PAF approximated. Thus, a classification improvement around 6% and 10% was reached by this classifier, respectively. In fact, the three considered patient groups were classified with accuracies of 95.42%, 79.29%, and 83.98%, respectively, the global accuracy being around 86%. Additionally, healthy subjects and PAF patients were discerned with an accuracy of 95.42% and false-positive rate around 5%.

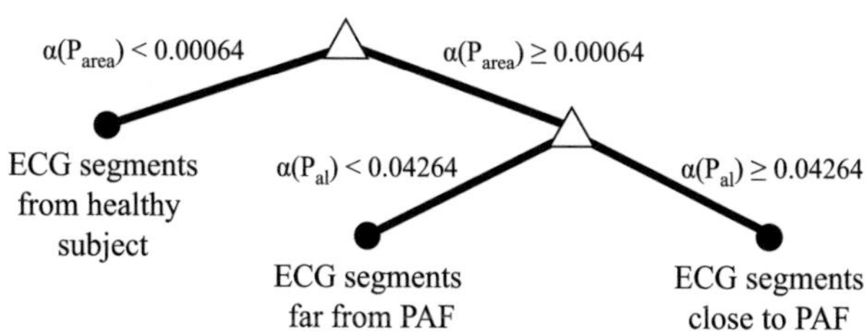

Figure 8. Decision tree generated from the learning sets to classify ECG segments from healthy subjects, far from PAF and close to PAF.

By considering these results, the analysis of the P-wave morphological variability over time could be considered as a useful tool to anticipate PAF. More concretely, the rectified P-wave length variability over time provided the highest statistical differences between groups of ECG segments and the best classification results from all the analyzed P-wave morphological features. As for the time P-wave features, higher morphological variability was observed when the onset of PAF approximated. This finding is in line with the atrial alterations preceding the onset of PAF, which eventually will provoke an intermittently disrupted electrical conduction [39].

Other authors have also suggested a greater P-wave morphology alteration when AF onset approximates. Thus, by using a P-wave modeling based on the addition of gaussian functions, more fragmented atrial depolarizations have been observed in patients with greater risk of AF development [15]. Similarly, the P-wave modeling based on singular value decomposition [60] or wavelet analysis [61] has also reported a higher P-wave complexity in patients developing AF after coronary artery bypass grafting compared to those who maintained normal sinus rhythm. Finally, making use of the P-wave spectral turbulence analysis, Barbosa et al. [62] have found a direct relationship between the probability of AF recurrence after electrical cardioversion and the P-wave fragmentation. However, it has to be remarked that such a kind of analysis was not proposed to study the beat-to-beat P-wave morphological alterations.

Regarding the P-wave energy, other works have reported higher energy values for PAF patients than for healthy subjects in the signal-averaged P-wave [17]. Similarly, within PAF patients, higher energy values have been observed in those patients with an increased number of episodes [16]. Moreover, a P-wave energy reduction after pharmacological treatment with antiarrhythmic drugs has also been corroborated by several authors [14]. Because these drugs can enlarge the refractory period without altering conduction velocity, this metric has been proposed as a noninvasive marker of atrial refractoriness [14]. According to this finding, parameters such as P_{area}, P_{nrms}, $P_{nenergy}$, and P_{narea} reported high variability over time. However, it is noteworthy that the P-wave energy has been computed in frequency [17] or wavelet [16] domains in the aforementioned previous work.

On the other hand, it is interesting to note that only the number of gaussian functions to appropriately fit this model to the signal-averaged P-wave was studied in [15]. Moreover, only spatial diversity between the acquired 32 leads was considered by comparing the obtained results from each other. Nonetheless, a similar P-wave modeling in a wave-to-wave fashion with a single gaussian function has also been proposed to analyze P-wave variability over time [27]. In order to quantify their morphology, each P-wave was modeled by a gaussian function defined as

$$\hat{w}[n] = A \cdot e^{-\left(\frac{n-C}{W}\right)^2}, \tag{18}$$

where the constants A, C, and W represent its amplitude, time position, and width, respectively. To compute these parameters, the gaussian function $\hat{w}[n]$ was fitted to every single P-wave by a nonlinear least squares approach [27].

On the other hand, previous works have proved that a normal P-wave resembles a gaussian shape [63]. However, altered and fractionated atrial electrical activity seems to be reflected in the appearance of bumps in the P-wave [15]. Therefore, higher differences between the real P-wave and its gaussian model could be expected when PAF onset approximates. This P-wave alteration can be assessed by the normalized root mean square error (ε) between the real and the gaussian modeled P-wave [27]. As an example, Fig. 9 shows typical cases of P-waves coming from healthy and diseased PAF patients together with their corresponding gaussian modeling. Observe how ε is able to represent quite robustly the differences between real and modeled P-waves.

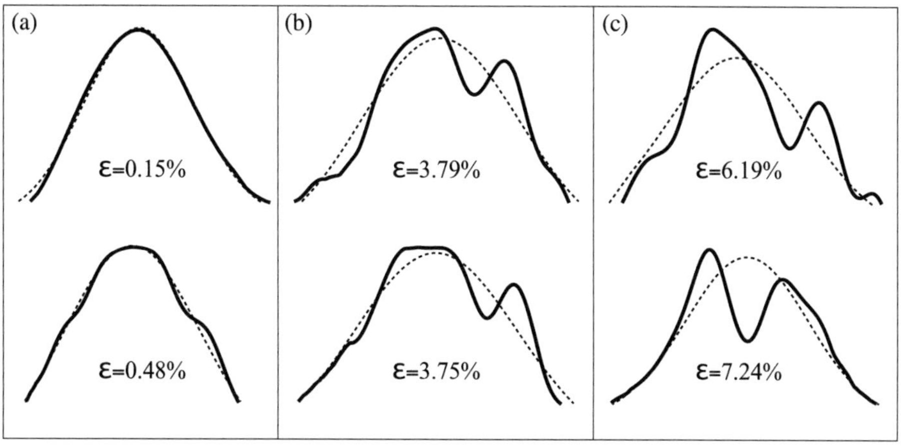

Figure 9. Comparison between the obtained gaussian models (dotted line) and representative P-waves (solid line) from typical (a) healthy subjects, (b) patients far from PAF, and (c) patients close to PAF. It has to be remarked that as PAF onset approximates, the root mean square error ε increases.

The variability of A, C, W, and ε over the one-hour-length recordings was estimated in the same way as before by fitting a linear model to the data in which the fitting slope (α) indicated the corresponding variability. The results obtained are summarized in Fig. 10. As was expected, an increased P-wave variability was shown by these parameters when the onset of PAF approximated. To this respect, the time course variability of W for typical ECG intervals from the studied groups is displayed in Fig. 11.

From a numerical point of view, the classification results are summarized in Table 3. As can be observed, parameters derived from the P-wave gaussian modeling did not improve the P_{dur} discriminant ability. However, the metric W only presented an accuracy slightly lower (around 3.5%) than the time course variability of the P-wave duration. In addition, a greater global accuracy than the feature PP_k was reached by the remaining morphological P-wave features. Thus, improvements around 3.5, 9, and 6% in the global accuracy were obtained from the metrics A, C, and ε, respectively, compared with the PP_k. Moreover, it is also interesting to note that a stepwise discriminant analysis provided a global accuracy increase of around 6 and 9% compared with the features P_{dur} and W, respectively. As expected, given that these metrics provided the highest single accuracy, they were combined to produce the optimal discriminant model.

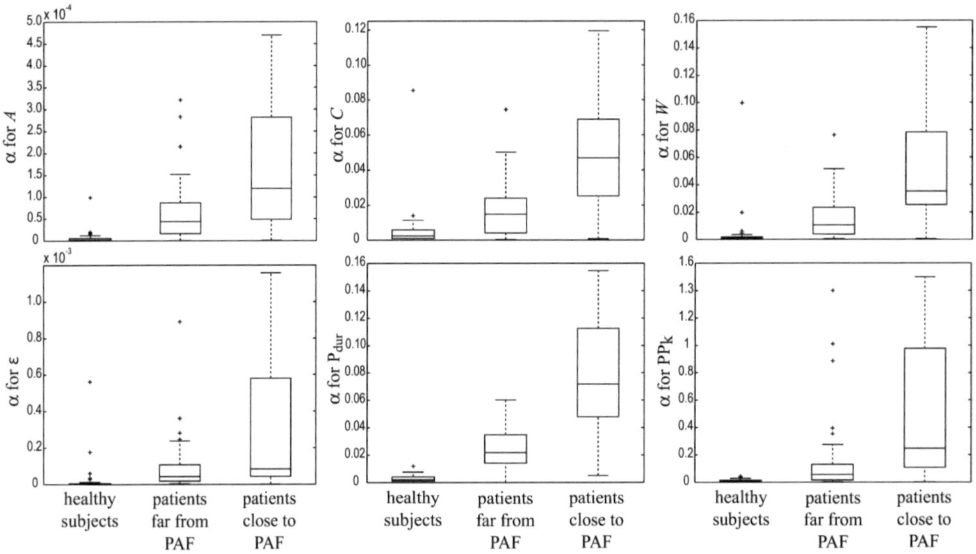

Figure 10. Boxplots showing the distribution of the fitting line slope associated to each analyzed parameter from the gaussian modeling of the P-wave for healthy subjects, patients far from PAF, and patients close to PAF.

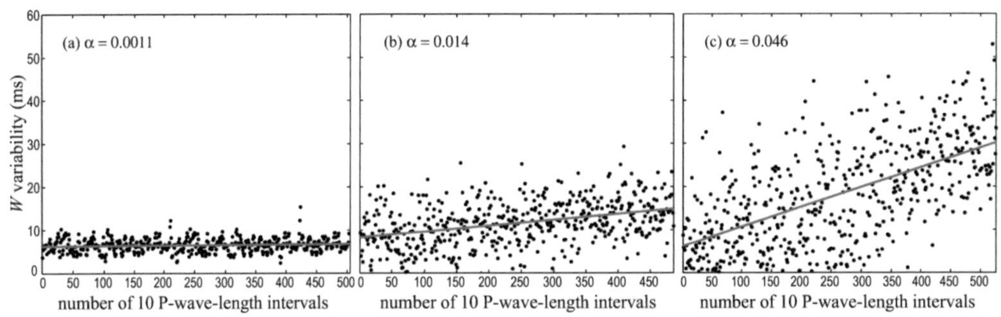

Figure 11. Typical P-wave width W variability over time from representative ECG intervals from (a) a healthy subject, (b) patients far from PAF, and (c) patients close to PAF.

Finally, it has to be remarked that other attempts to quantify the P-wave morphology can also be found in the literature. To this respect, a classification rate higher than 90% among P-waves with different morphologies has been reached by means of systems identification in [64]. On the other hand, the AF risk after post-coronary artery bypass grafting has been successfully quantified by analyzing the singular value decomposition of the P-wave morphology [60]. Similarly, Clavier et al. [24] have presented an automatic method based on a hidden Markov model and wavelet transform to detect and delineate the P-wave. Moreover, they also proposed a polynomial characterization of this wave, thus noticing the need of higher orders to represent slight morphological details of the P-wave. Finally, the P-wave energy has also been analyzed by several authors from wavelet and frequency domains [16, 17], providing P-waves with higher energy when the risk of AF development was increased.

Feature	Healthy subjects		Far from PAF		Close to PAF		Global Accuracy	
	training	test	training	test	training	test	training	test
A	85.79%	82.16%	59.78%	47.83%	67.39%	59.78%	71.74%	66.16%
C	86.78%	81.84%	60.65%	53.91%	78.70%	74.78%	75.92%	71.75%
W	89.64%	86.91%	75.87%	64.13%	82.43%	78.30%	83.19%	77.36%
ε	84.92%	77.12%	58.91%	49.13%	71.96%	67.83%	72.55%	68.30%
P_{dur}	93.88%	91.47%	80.61%	69.58%	85.17%	80.42%	88.90%	81.02%
PP_k	85.24%	78.17%	48.04%	37.39%	73.70%	69.78%	69.78%	62.54%

Table 3. Percentage of ECG segments correctly classified for each group from the slope α obtained for each studied P-wave feature from its gaussian modeling.

4. Spatial analysis of the P-wave

The P-wave duration has also been widely characterized from the standard 12-lead ECG recording. Thus, the P-wave duration has been normally measured in at least ten of the 12 surface leads, with the maximum being the longest P-wave duration in any lead and the minimum being the shortest P-wave duration in any lead [38]. Moreover, the P-wave dispersion has been defined as the difference between the maximum and the minimum P-wave duration [39]. Whereas the minimum P-wave duration has only provided recently significant clinical information to identify an increased risk of lone AF [65], the maximum one and its dispersion have shown to be widely useful in the prediction of PAF. To this respect, Dilaveris et al. [38] found a high correlation between the maximum P-wave duration and the risk of idiopathic PAF. Moreover, the P-wave dispersion complemented this metric for a clearer separation between patients with PAF and normal controls. These findings were validated two years later by Aytemir et al. [47], who analyzed a slightly wider database. Additionally, De Bacquer et al. [66] showed that the maximum P-wave duration was a very important risk indicator for the development of AF over 10 years. In agreement with these works, Andrikopoulos et al. [67] showed that the maximum P-wave duration and its dispersion were significantly higher in patients with PAF than in control subjects. However, these authors also reported that the variance of the P-wave duration in the 12-lead ECG was a stronger predictor of the onset of idiopathic PAF than the previous metrics. The same result was also obtained by Perez et al. [40], who measured the standard deviation of the P-wave in the ECG. However, in this case, more than 40,000 patients who were followed for the development of AF for at least 5 years were analyzed. In view of this outcome, the authors suggested that the P-wave variance may account for the differences in atrial conduction across different areas, thus reflecting more accurately the heterogeneity of the diseased atria.

In addition to these works, others have also corroborated the usefulness of the P-wave dispersion to predict the onset of PAF. Thus, Dilaveris et al. [68] showed the ability of this metric to predict frequent symptomatic AF paroxysms. In the same study, a significant positive correlation was observed between the P-wave dispersion and its maximum duration. Similarly, a relevant negative correlation was noticed between the P-wave dispersion and its minimum duration. In another publication, the P-wave dispersion also showed to be a sensitive and specific ECG predictor of paroxysmal lone AF. Furthermore, it also provided a significant correlation with the maximum P-wave duration and a weak, although significant, association with age [47]. On the other hand, Dilaveris et al. [69] and Ciaroni et al. [70] revealed the P-wave dispersion as an independent predictor of the onset of PAF in the hypertensive population. Indeed, this metric was found to be significantly higher in hypertensives with a history of PAF than those without history of arrhythmia. Finally, it is interesting to mention that Koide et al. [71] concluded that the P-wave dispersion was a clinically useful predictor of progression from paroxysmal to persistent AF. In this study, more than 200 patients with a diagnosis of PAF were followed for more than 60 months.

5. Discussion

Recent works have shown that the beat-to-beat analysis of the P-wave can reveal clinically relevant information about the altered atrial conduction preceding the onset of PAF as any signal-averaging approach. Furthermore, the main advantage of the individualized single P-wave analysis is the possibility of being easily used in a routine clinical environment, because it can be developed from daily recordings such as short surface ECGs or long-term Holter signals. Hence, this kind of P-wave analysis could be considered as the most practical way to perform exploratory investigations about the onset of PAF.

It is highly relevant to highlight that in recent years, the analysis of PAC has been improved to reach a clinically significant result. Thus, it has been able to identify the imminent onset of PAF with an accuracy very near to 100%. However, it has also been noticed that the frequency of these ectopics is considerably decreased as the distance to the episode onset increases [53, 52]. Therefore, it could be elucidated that this approach is only feasible just before the arrhythmia starts [31], which is too late for the application of an efficient prophylactic therapy [72, 73]. In contrast, the analysis of the P-wave variability over time has proven to be able to operate with notably more anticipation in the prediction of PAF onset. Indeed, the time evolution of all the studied P-wave features has revealed an interesting ability to predict successfully the onset of PAF with, at least, one hour in advance.

Moreover, it is worth noting that all the analyzed P-wave features show a time course variation as a function of how far is the onset of PAF. Indeed, all the analyzed features provided an increased variability trend as the PAF onset approximates. This outcome is in strong agreement with the atrial electrophysiological alterations noticed in clinical studies before the onset of spontaneous or induced AF. To this respect, a common atrial alteration in patients prone to PAF is the presence of decreased and different cell refractory periods in various atrial regions. Sometimes, these site-specific conduction delays can be increased by intracellular or intercellular factors, such as connections, ion channels, or regulatory proteins [9, 74]. This heterogeneity may provoke irregular atrial conduction which could result in overlapped atrial depolarizations or even premature atrial repolarizations [42, 2]. Thus, the way through which the sinus beat travels across the atria may be notably altered by the presence of these delays as well as structural abnormalities in atrial walls (e.g., fibrosis) [9]. Hence, the highly variable and fragmented atrial activation morphology over time could be a result from this site-dependent inhomogeneous and intermittent atrial conduction [39]. Overall, the beat-to-beat analysis to quantify P-wave progression over time seems to be a promising new way to identify the onset of PAF. Furthermore, the study about how this method's performance is maintained in more anticipated predictions has to be validated in future prospective studies. In this way, earlier predictions of the onset of PAF could be reached and patients could benefit from preventive therapies.

Finally, although the single P-wave analysis from short ECGs cannot provide information about the time progression of the atrial electrophysiological alterations preceding the onset of PAF, it can reveal interesting information about the regional differences in atrial activation and conduction [39]. To this respect, previous works have shown that the electrical activity in the surface ECG closely correlates with the conduction in specific parts of the atria [75]. Hence, inhomogeneous atrial conduction can be identified by variations in the P-wave duration between differently oriented surface ECG leads [39]. This information has proven to be widely useful to discern between PAF patients and healthy subjects from the sinus rhythm ECG. This is also an interesting clinical challenge [32] because PAF can sometimes be asymptomatic and not only a single episode may appear during long-time Holter monitoring. Thus, this information could allow the identification of patients with PAF without the need of long-term recordings and they may be early treated, thus minimizing the atrial remodeling and reducing the probability of arrhythmia perpetuation.

6. Conclusions

This study aimed to review the most recent advances in the beat-to-beat P-wave analysis to stratify the risk of suffering PAF and how long in advance its onset can be predicted. In recent years, considerable progress has been reached in both purposes, this kind of analysis being able to provide, in an easy and noninvasive way, clinically useful information related to the time progression and regional differences of the atrial conduction alterations preceding the onset of PAF. The use of this information may be helpful in routine clinical practice to improve the diagnostic and therapeutic management of atrial fibrillation.

Acknowledgements

This work was supported by the projects TEC2014-52250-R from the Spanish Ministry of Economy and Competitiveness and PPII-2014-026-P from Junta de Comunidades de Castilla La Mancha.

Author details

Raúl Alcaraz[1*] and José Joaquín Rieta[2]

*Address all correspondence to: raul.alcaraz@uclm.es

1 Innovation in Bioengineering Research Group, University of Castilla-La Mancha, Cuenca, Spain

2 Biomedical Synergy, Electronic Engineering Department, Universidad Politécnica de Valencia, Gandia, Spain

References

[1] Rich MW. Epidemiology of atrial fibrillation. J Interv Card Electrophysiol Jun 2009;25(1):3–8.

[2] American College of Cardiology Foundation, American Heart Association, European Society of Cardiology, Heart Rhythm Society, Wann LS, Curtis AB, Ellenbogen KA, Estes NAM, Ezekowitz MD, Jackman WM, January CT, Lowe JE, Page RL, Slotwiner DJ, Stevenson WG, Tracy CM, Fuster V, Rydén LE, Cannom DS, Crijns HJ, Curtis AB, Ellenbogen KA, Halperin JL, Le Heuzey JY, Kay GN, Lowe JE, Olsson SB, Prystowsky EN, Tamargo JL, Wann LS. Management of patients with atrial fibrillation (compilation of 2006 ACCF/AHA/ESC and 2011 ACCF/AHA/HRS recommendations): a report of the American College of Cardiology/American Heart Association Task Force on practice guidelines. Circulation May 2013;127(18):1916–26.

[3] Gallagher MM, Camm J. Classification of atrial fibrillation. Am J Cardiol Oct 1998;82(8A):18N–28N.

[4] de Vos CB, Pisters R, Nieuwlaat R, Prins MH, Tieleman RG, Coelen RJS, van den Heijkant AC, Allessie MA, Crijns HJGM. Progression from paroxysmal to persistent atrial fibrillation clinical correlates and prognosis. J Am Coll Cardiol Feb 2010;55(8): 725–31.

[5] Petrutiu S, Sahakian AV, Swiryn S. Abrupt changes in fibrillatory wave characteristics at the termination of paroxysmal atrial fibrillation in humans. Europace Jul 2007;9(7):466–70.

[6] Prystowsky EN. Management of atrial fibrillation: therapeutic options and clinical decisions. Am J Cardiol May 2000;85(10A):3D–11D.

[7] Dilaveris PE, Gialafos JE. Future concepts in P wave morphological analyses. Card Electrophysiol Rev Sep 2002;6(3):221–4.

[8] Platonov PG, Carlson J, Ingemansson MP, Roijer A, Hansson A, Chireikin LV, Olsson SB. Detection of inter-atrial conduction defects with unfiltered signal-averaged p-wave ecg in patients with lone atrial fibrillation. Europace Jan 2000;2(1):32–41.

[9] Platonov PG. P-wave morphology: underlying mechanisms and clinical implications. Ann Noninvasive Electrocardiol Jul 2012;17(3):161–9.

[10] Magnani JW, Zhu L, Lopez F, Pencina MJ, Agarwal SK, Soliman EZ, Benjamin EJ, Alonso A. P-wave indices and atrial fibrillation: cross-cohort assessments from the framingham heart study (fhs) and atherosclerosis risk in communities (aric) study. Am Heart J Jan 2015;169(1):53–61.e1.

[11] Platonov PG. Atrial conduction and atrial fibrillation: what can we learn from surface ECG? Cardiol J 2008;15(5):402–7.

[12] Dilaveris P, Stefanadis C. Current morphologic and vectorial aspects of p-wave analysis. J Electrocardiol 2009;42(5):395–9.

[13] Censi F, Ricci C, Calcagnini G, Triventi M, Ricci RP, Santini M, Bartolini P. Time-domain and morphological analysis of the P-wave. Part I: technical aspects for automatic quantification of P-wave features. Pacing Clin Electrophysiol Jul 2008;31(7):874–83.

[14] Stafford PJ, Kamalvand K, Tan K, Vincent R, Sulke N. Prediction of maintenance of sinus rhythm after cardioversion of atrial fibrillation by analysis of serial signal-averaged p waves. Pacing Clin Electrophysiol Jul 1998;21(7):1387–95.

[15] Censi F, Calcagnini G, Ricci C, Ricci RP, Santini M, Grammatico A, Bartolini P. P-wave morphology assessment by a gaussian functions-based model in atrial fibrillation patients. IEEE Trans Biomed Eng Apr 2007;54(4):663–72.

[16] Vassilikos V, Dakos G, Chatzizisis YS, Chouvarda I, Karvounis C, Maynard C, Maglaveras N, Paraskevaidis S, Stavropoulos G, Styliadis CI, Mochlas S, Styliadis I. Novel non-invasive P wave analysis for the prediction of paroxysmal atrial fibrillation recurrences in patients without structural heart disease: a prospective pilot study. Int J Cardiol Dec 2011;153(2):165–72.

[17] Stafford PJ, Robinson D, Vincent R. Optimal analysis of the signal averaged P wave in patients with paroxysmal atrial fibrillation. Br Heart J Oct 1995;74(4):413–8.

[18] Blanche C, Tran N, Rigamonti F, Burri H, Zimmermann M. Value of p-wave signal averaging to predict atrial fibrillation recurrences after pulmonary vein isolation. Europace Feb 2013;15(2):198–204.

[19] Masuda M, Inoue K, Iwakura K, Okamura A, Toyoshima Y, Doi A, Sotomi Y, Komuro I, Fujii K. Impact of pulmonary vein isolation on atrial late potentials: association with the recurrence of atrial fibrillation. Europace Apr 2013;15(4):501–7.

[20] Hayashida N, Shojima T, Yokokura Y, Hori H, Yoshikawa K, Tomoeda H, Aoyagi S. P-wave signal-averaged electrocardiogram for predicting atrial arrhythmia after cardiac surgery. Ann Thorac Surg Mar 2005;79(3):859–64.

[21] Gonna H, Gallagher MM, Guo XH, Yap YG, Hnatkova K, Camm AJ. P-wave abnormality predicts recurrence of atrial fibrillation after electrical cardioversion: a prospective study. Ann Noninvasive Electrocardiol Jan 2014;19(1):57–62.

[22] Ros E, Mota S, Fernández FJ, Toro FJ, Bernier JL. ECG characterization of paroxysmal atrial fibrillation: parameter extraction and automatic diagnosis algorithm. Comput Biol Med Dec 2004;34(8):679–96.

[23] Hayn D, Kollmann A, Schreier G. Predicting initiation and termination of atrial fibrillation from the ecg. Biomed Tech Berl Feb 2007;52(1):5–10.

[24] Clavier L, Boucher JM, Lepage R, Blanc JJ, Cornily JC. Automatic P-wave analysis of patients prone to atrial fibrillation. Med Biol Eng Comput Jan 2002;40(1):63–71.

[25] Martnez A, Alcaraz R, Rieta JJ. Study on the p-wave feature time course as early predictors of paroxysmal atrial fibrillation. Physiol Meas Dec 2012;33(12):1959–74.

[26] Martnez A, Alcaraz R, Rieta JJ. Morphological variability of the p-wave for premature envision of paroxysmal atrial fibrillation events. Physiol Meas Jan 2014;35(1):1–14.

[27] Martnez A, Alcaraz R, Rieta JJ. Gaussian modeling of the p-wave morphology time course applied to anticipate paroxysmal atrial fibrillation. Comput Methods Biomech Biomed Eng Oct 2014;1–10.

[28] Hassaguerre M, Jas P, Shah DC, Takahashi A, Hocini M, Quiniou G, Garrigue S, Mouroux AL, Métayer PL, Clémenty J. Spontaneous initiation of atrial fibrillation by ectopic beats originating in the pulmonary veins. N Engl J Med Sep 1998;339(10):659–666.

[29] Tsai CF, Tai CT, Hsieh MH, Lin WS, Yu WC, Ueng KC, Ding YA, Chang MS, Chen SA. Initiation of atrial fibrillation by ectopic beats originating from the superior vena cava: electrophysiological characteristics and results of radiofrequency ablation. Circulation Jul 2000;102(1):67–74.

[30] Kolb C, Nürnberger S, Ndrepepa G, Zrenner B, Schömig A, Schmitt C. Modes of initiation of paroxysmal atrial fibrillation from analysis of spontaneously occurring episodes using a 12-lead holter monitoring system. Am J Cardiol Oct 2001;88(8):853–7.

[31] Thong T, McNames J, Aboy M, Goldstein B. Prediction of paroxysmal atrial fibrillation by analysis of atrial premature complexes. IEEE Trans Biomed Eng Apr 2004;51(4):561–9.

[32] Hickey B, Heneghan C, de Chazal P. Non-episode-dependent assessment of paroxysmal atrial fibrillation through measurement of RR interval dynamics and atrial premature contractions. Ann Biomed Eng May 2004;32(5):677–87.

[33] Goldberger AL, Amaral LA, Glass L, Hausdorff JM, Ivanov PC, Mark RG, Mietus JE, Moody GB, Peng CK, Stanley HE. Physiobank, physiotoolkit, and physionet: components of a new research resource for complex physiologic signals. Circulation Jun 2000;101(23):E215–20.

[34] Langley P, Di Bernardo D, Allen J, Bowers E, Smith F, Vecchietti S, Murray A. Can paroxysmal atrial fibrillation be predicted? Comput Cardiol 2001;28:121–4.

[35] Zhong W, Mukkamala R, Mark R. A methodology for predicting paroxysmal atrial fibrillation based on ECG arrhythmia feature analysis. Comput Cardiol 2001;28:125–8.

[36] Schreier G, Kaster P, Marko W. An automatic EGC processing algorithm to identify patients prone to paroxysmal atrial fibrillation. Comput Cardiol 2001;28:133–5.

[37] Martnez A, Alcaraz R, Rieta JJ. Application of the phasor transform for automatic delineation of single-lead ECG fiducial points. Physiol Meas Nov 2010;31(11):1467–85.

[38] Dilaveris PE, Gialafos EJ, Sideris SK, Theopistou AM, Andrikopoulos GK, Kyriakidis M, Gialafos JE, Toutouzas PK. Simple electrocardiographic markers for the prediction of paroxysmal idiopathic atrial fibrillation. Am Heart J May 1998;135(5 Pt 1):733–8.

[39] Dilaveris PE, Gialafos JE. P-wave dispersion: a novel predictor of paroxysmal atrial fibrillation. Ann Noninvasive Electrocardiol Apr 2001;6(2):159–65.

[40] Perez MV, Dewey FE, Marcus R, Ashley EA, Al-Ahmad AA, Wang PJ, Froelicher VF. Electrocardiographic predictors of atrial fibrillation. Am Heart J Oct 2009;158(4):622–8.

[41] Ishida K, Hayashi H, Miyamoto A, Sugimoto Y, Ito M, Murakami Y, Horie M. P wave and the development of atrial fibrillation. Heart Rhythm Mar 2010;7(3):289–94.

[42] Sovilj S, Van Oosterom A, Rajsman G, Magjarevic R. ECG-based prediction of atrial fibrillation development following coronary artery bypass grafting. Physiol Meas May 2010;31(5):663–77.

[43] Cheng S, Keyes MJ, Larson MG, McCabe EL, Newton-Cheh C, Levy D, Benjamin EJ, Vasan RS, Wang TJ. Long-term outcomes in individuals with prolonged PR interval or first-degree atrioventricular block. JAMA Jun 2009;301(24):2571–7.

[44] Schnabel RB, Sullivan LM, Levy D, Pencina MJ, Massaro JM, D'Agostino Sr RB, Newton-Cheh C, Yamamoto JF, Magnani JW, Tadros TM, Kannel WB, Wang TJ, Ellinor PT, Wolf PA, Vasan RS, Benjamin EJ. Development of a risk score for atrial fibrilla-

tion (framingham heart study): a community-based cohort study. Lancet Feb 2009;373(9665):739–45.

[45] Uhley H. Determination of risk for atrial fibrillation utilizing precise P wave duration-measuring methodology. Prev Cardiol 2001;4(2):81–3.

[46] Magnani JW, Mazzini MJ, Sullivan LM, Williamson M, Ellinor PT, Benjamin EJ. P-wave indices, distribution and quality control assessment (from the framingham heart study). Ann Noninvasive Electrocardiol Jan 2010;15(1):77–84.

[47] Aytemir K, Ozer N, Atalar E, Sade E, Aksöyek S, Ovünç K, Oto A, Ozmen F, Kes S. P wave dispersion on 12-lead electrocardiography in patients with paroxysmal atrial fibrillation. Pacing Clin Electrophysiol Jul 2000;23(7):1109–12.

[48] Liu Z, Hayano M, Hirata T, Quin Y, Tsukahara K, Ishimatsu T, Sakamoto R, Iliev I, Iwamoto K, Ueyama C, Yano K. Abnormalities of electrocardiographic P wave morphology and the relationship to electrophysiological parameters of the atrium in patients with idiopathic paroxysmal atrial fibrillation. J Cardiol Sep 1998;32(3):189–96.

[49] Poli S, Barbaro V, Bartolini P, Calcagnini G, Censi F. Prediction of atrial fibrillation from surface ECG: review of methods and algorithms. Ann Ist Super Sanita Jan 2003;39(2):195–203.

[50] Cabasson A, Dang L, Vesin J, Buttu A, Abächerli R, Leber R, Kappenberger L. P-wave indices to detect susceptibility to atrial fibrillation. Comput Cardiol 2011;257–60.

[51] Passman R, Beshai J, Pavri B, Kimmel S. Predicting post-coronary bypass surgery atrial arrhythmias from the preoperative electrocardiogram. Am Heart J Nov 2001;142(5):806–10.

[52] Vikman S, Mäkikallio TH, Yli-Mäyry S, Pikkujämsä S, Koivisto AM, Reinikainen P, Airaksinen KE, Huikuri HV. Altered complexity and correlation properties of R-R interval dynamics before the spontaneous onset of paroxysmal atrial fibrillation. Circulation Nov 1999;100(20):2079–84.

[53] Shin DG, Yoo CS, Yi SH, Bae JH, Kim YJ, Park JS, Hong GR. Prediction of paroxysmal atrial fibrillation using nonlinear analysis of the R-R interval dynamics before the spontaneous onset of atrial fibrillation. Circ J Jan 2006;70(1):94–9.

[54] Tuzcu V, Nas S, Börklü T, Ugur A. Decrease in the heart rate complexity prior to the onset of atrial fibrillation. Europace Jun 2006;8(6):398–402.

[55] Chesnokov YV. Complexity and spectral analysis of the heart rate variability dynamics for distant prediction of paroxysmal atrial fibrillation with artificial intelligence methods. Artif Intell Med Jun 2008;43(2):151–65.

[56] Mohebbi M, Ghassemian H. Prediction of paroxysmal atrial fibrillation based on non-linear analysis and spectrum and bispectrum features of the heart rate variability signal. Comput Methods Programs Biomed Jan 2012;105(1):40–9.

[57] Mohebbi M, Ghassemian H. Prediction of paroxysmal atrial fibrillation using recurrence plot-based features of the RR-interval signal. Physiol Meas Aug 2011;32(8): 1147–62.

[58] Molina-Picó A, Cuesta-Frau D, Aboy M, Crespo C, Miró-Martnez P, Oltra-Crespo S. Comparative study of approximate entropy and sample entropy robustness to spikes. Artif Intell Med Oct 2011;53(2):97–106.

[59] Van Beeumen K, Houben R, Tavernier R, Ketels S, Duytschaever M. Changes in P-wave area and P-wave duration after circumferential pulmonary vein isolation. Europace Jun 2010;12(6):798–804.

[60] Gang Y, Hnatkova K, Mandal K, Ghuran A, Malik M. Preoperative electrocardiographic risk assessment of atrial fibrillation after coronary artery bypass grafting. J Cardiovasc Electrophysiol Dec 2004;15(12):1379–86.

[61] Vassilikos V, Dakos G, Chouvarda I, Karagounis L, Karvounis H, Maglaveras N, Mochlas S, Spanos P, Louridas G. Can P wave wavelet analysis predict atrial fibrillation after coronary artery bypass grafting? Pacing Clin Electrophysiol Jan 2003;26(1 Pt 2): 305–9.

[62] Benchimol-Barbosa PR, de Souza-Bomfim A, Barbosa EC, Ginefra P, Helena Cardoso Boghossian S, Destro C, Nadal J. Spectral turbulence analysis of the signal-averaged electrocardiogram of the atrial activation as predictor of recurrence of idiopathic and persistent atrial fibrillation. Int J Cardiol Mar 2006;107(3):307–16.

[63] Dubois R, Maison-Blanche P, Quenet B, Dreyfus G. Automatic ECG wave extraction in long-term recordings using Gaussian mesa function models and nonlinear probability estimators. Comput Methods Programs Biomed Dec 2007;88(3):217–33.

[64] Carlson J, Johansson R, Olsson SB. Classification of electrocardiographic P-wave morphology. IEEE Trans Biomed Eng Apr 2001;48(4):401–5.

[65] Chang ICY, Austin E, Krishnan B, Benditt DG, Quay CN, Ling LH, Chen LY. Shorter minimum p-wave duration is associated with paroxysmal lone atrial fibrillation. J Electrocardiol 2014;47(1):106–12.

[66] De Bacquer D, Willekens J, De Backer G. Long-term prognostic value of P-wave characteristics for the development of atrial fibrillation in subjects aged 55 to 74 years at baseline. Am J Cardiol Sep 2007;100(5):850–4.

[67] Andrikopoulos GK, Dilaveris PE, Richter DJ, Gialafos EJ, Synetos AG, Gialafos JE. Increased variance of P wave duration on the electrocardiogram distinguishes patients with idiopathic paroxysmal atrial fibrillation. Pacing Clin Electrophysiol Jul 2000;23(7):1127–32.

[68] Dilaveris PE, Gialafos EJ, Andrikopoulos GK, Richter DJ, Papanikolaou V, Poralis K, Gialafos JE. Clinical and electrocardiographic predictors of recurrent atrial fibrillation. Pacing Clin Electrophysiol Mar 2000;23(3):352–8.

[69] Dilaveris PE, Gialafos EJ, Chrissos D, Andrikopoulos GK, Richter DJ, Lazaki E, Gialafos JE. Detection of hypertensive patients at risk for paroxysmal atrial fibrillation during sinus rhythm by computer-assisted p wave analysis. J Hypertens Oct 1999;17(10):1463–70.

[70] Ciaroni S, Cuenoud L, Bloch A. Clinical study to investigate the predictive parameters for the onset of atrial fibrillation in patients with essential hypertension. Am Heart J May 2000;139(5):814–9.

[71] Koide Y, Yotsukura M, Ando H, Aoki S, Suzuki T, Sakata K, Ootomo E, Yoshino H. Usefulness of p-wave dispersion in standard twelve-lead electrocardiography to predict transition from paroxysmal to persistent atrial fibrillation. Am J Cardiol Sep 2008;102(5):573–7.

[72] Dimmer C, Tavernier R, Gjorgov N, Van Nooten G, Clement DL, Jordaens L. Variations of autonomic tone preceding onset of atrial fibrillation after coronary artery bypass grafting. Am J Cardiol Jul 1998;82(1):22–5.

[73] Hogue Jr CW, Domitrovich PP, Stein PK, Despotis GD, Re L, Schuessler RB, Kleiger RE, Rottman JN. RR interval dynamics before atrial fibrillation in patients after coronary artery bypass graft surgery. Circulation Aug 1998;98(5):429–34.

[74] Papageorgiou P, Monahan K, Boyle NG, Seifert MJ, Beswick P, Zebede J, Epstein LM, Josephson ME. Site-dependent intra-atrial conduction delay. Relationship to initiation of atrial fibrillation. Circulation Aug 1996;94(3):384–9.

[75] Ndrepepa G, Zrenner B, Deisenhofer I, Karch M, Schneider M, Schreieck J, Schmitt C. Relationship between surface electrocardiogram characteristics and endocardial activation sequence in patients with typical atrial flutter. Z Kardiol Jun 2000;89(6):527–37.

Chapter 3

Clinical Significance of Arrhythmogenic Foci in Atrial Fibrillation

Toshiya Kurotobi

Additional information is available at the end of the chapter

http://dx.doi.org/10.5772/60646

Abstract

Atrial fibrillation (AF) is initiated by pulmonary vein (PV) and non-PV foci, which could be associated with initiating and maintaining AF. The development of the remodeling process and preexistent anatomical structures are likely to relate to the structural and electrophysiological changes in the PVs and non-PV area, which could promote the local conduction abnormalities and cause an increased PV/non-PV arrhythmogenicity. In this section, we assessed the features and relating factors of PV/non-PV arrhythmogenicity in patients with AF and evaluated its clinical implication. As a result, we realized the atrial anatomical features, such as the left atrial roof shape, left lateral ridge, and Marshall vein provided us with an understanding of PV and non-PV arrhythmogenicity in patients with AF. In addition, the presence of residual arrhythmogenic non-PV foci is associated with increased AF recurrence after catheter ablation; therefore, the information of arrhythmogenic foci (AMF) is also useful for determining the appropriate strategy of ablation for AF.

Keywords: atrial fibrillation, catheter ablation, arrhythmogenic foci, structural remodeling, Marshall bundle

1. Introduction

Atrial fibrillation (AF) is caused by triggers from pulmonary veins (PVs) [1], and a rapid firing from the PVs could be responsible for initiating and maintaining arrhythmias in patients with

AF. The enhanced automaticity or triggered activity mechanisms could be involved in the initiation of AF [2, 3]. In addition, the PV's circumference is also most likely crucial for sustaining the reentry of maintaining AF [4], which can enhance a condition for persistent AF.

Non-PV foci can also arise from the crista terminalis, ostium of the coronary sinus, interatrial septum, superior vena cava, left atrial posterior free wall, and Marshall bundle [5, 6] with the incidence ranging from 3.2 to 47 % [7, 8, 9]. The dominant triggering sites of non-PV have a slow diastolic depolarization, increasing the chance of the spontaneous depolarization [10], and the triggered activity from the non-PV sites could also be involved in the initiation and perpetuation of AF. Previous studies have reported that the increased delay after depolarizations has been documented from the superior vena cava [10], coronary sinus (CS) [11], Marshall bundle and the coronary sinus [12], atrial muscle that extends into the mitral valve [13], and working muscle [14]. Especially, the Marshall bundle may be a crucial structure to initiate catecholamine-sensitive AF.

The development of the remodeling process and preexistent anatomical structures seems to be related to the structural and electrophysiological remodeling in the PVs and atrium, which can increase the local abnormal conduction and develop an increased PV/non-PV arrhythmogenicity leading to AF persistency [15, 16, 17, 10, 11].

In this section, we assessed the features and relating factors of PV/non-PV arrhythmogenicity in patients with AF and evaluated their clinical implication during catheter ablation procedure.

2. The feature and clinical implication of arrhythmogenic foci of atrial fibrillation

2.1. The method of induction and detection of PV/non-PV arrhythmogenic foci

We used five multipolar catheters recording the electrograms to search for the location of the arrhythmogenic foci (AMF). A 20-pole catheter covered the SVC to the crista terminalis, CS, and the left PVs. A mapping catheter was located at the right superior PV (Figure 1). When the AMF have originated from a non-PV area uncovered by the catheters, we searched the location with a mapping catheter. The 12-lead ECG and intracardiac electrograms were filtered between 30 to 500 Hz (DUO EP Laboratory; Bard Electrophysiology, Lowell, MA, USA).

The occurrence of PV/non-PV foci could be influenced by the induction methods, and PV arrhythmogenicity may be enhanced by the stimulation with acetylcholine or isoproterenol (ISP) [2, 18]. The relationship between the ISP dose and arrhythmogenicity remains unclear; however, the PV/non-PV foci are likely to be revealed with a high-dose isoproterenol up to 20 g/min or subsequent cardioversion of AF [19, 20]. High-dose ISP can cause the vagally mediated nerve reflex bradycardia, which seems to increase arrhythmogenicity after autonomic nerve competition.

Both atrial spontaneous AMF were carefully searched before the PV isolation procedure under an intravenous infusion of isoproterenol (ISP) without sedation. During sinus rhythm, ISP was

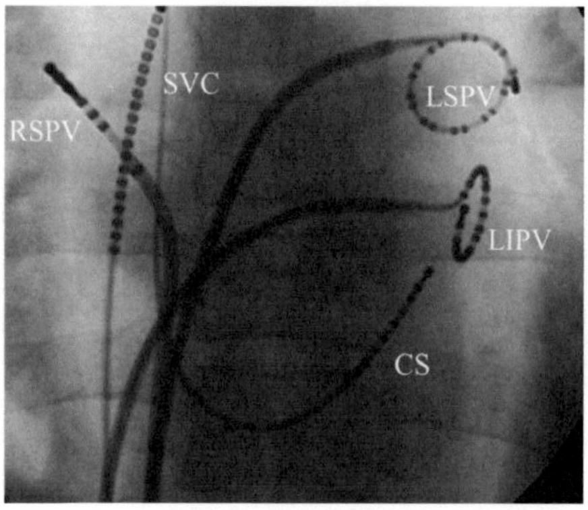

LSPV, left superior pulmonary vein; LIPV, left inferior pulmonary vein; CS, coronary sinus; RSPV, right superior pulmonary vein; SVC, superior vena cava.

Figure 1. Catheter locations for detecting AMF. Twenty-pole circular catheters were positioned at the left superior and inferior PV. A 10- or 20-pole catheter was located in the CS, and then terminal crest and the SVC were covered with a 20-pole catheter. The mapping catheter was located at the RSPV. When arrhythmogenic foci arise from the RIPV or a non-PV area, the suspected area was confirmed by a mapping catheter. The location of the PV/non-PV foci showing the earliest atrial focus was referred to the local electrogram or onset of the ectopic P wave. In addition, the direction of the earliest activated site of the PV/non-PV foci could be also determined by the sequence of the activation recorded from multipolar catheters allowing to detect the non-PV sites in both atria.

initially delivered at 1–2 g/min for 5 min, and then the dose was gradually increased up to 20 g/min with careful monitoring of the blood pressure. When the blood pressure dropped under 70 mm Hg, the dose of ISP was reversed to the basal level. When AF persisted and/or spontaneously occurred, direct cardioversion (DC) was attempted up to three times. The DC energy was delivered by using an external biphasic wave up to 270 J, and sinus rhythm was temporarily or successfully restored in all enrolled patients.

The ISP administration was maintained at basal level (1–2 g/min) during the ablation. At the end of the session, the increased dose of ISP was administered up to 20 g/min. AMF were confirmed as direct AF triggers and/or reproducible atrial premature beats with coupling intervals of <350 ms or frequent firings (Figure 2).

2.2. The location of PV/non-PV arrhythmogenic foci

Two hundred fourteen consecutive patients with drug-refractory AF episodes were enrolled in this study (mean age of 61 years, male, 71 %; persistent AF, 21%). The clinical and electrophysiologic characteristics of the AMF were demonstrated in Figure 3. Five hundred AMF were observed. PV and/or non-PV foci were detected in 201 of 214 (93.9 %). Two hundred sixty-three foci (52.6 %) in 174 patients (81.3 %) were confirmed as the triggers directly shifted to AF, and 237 foci (47.4 %) in 150 patients (70.1 %) showed reproducible premature atrial beats with an interval of <350 ms or repetitive firings. PV foci were confirmed in 195 of 214 patients (91 %) and non-PV foci in 107 of 214 (50 %), accounting for one third of all the AMF. Foci originating from only PVs were detected in 95 of 214 patients (44 %), both PV and non-PV origins in 98 of 214 (46 %), and only non-PV origins in 8 of 214 (3.7 %). Non-PV foci are located

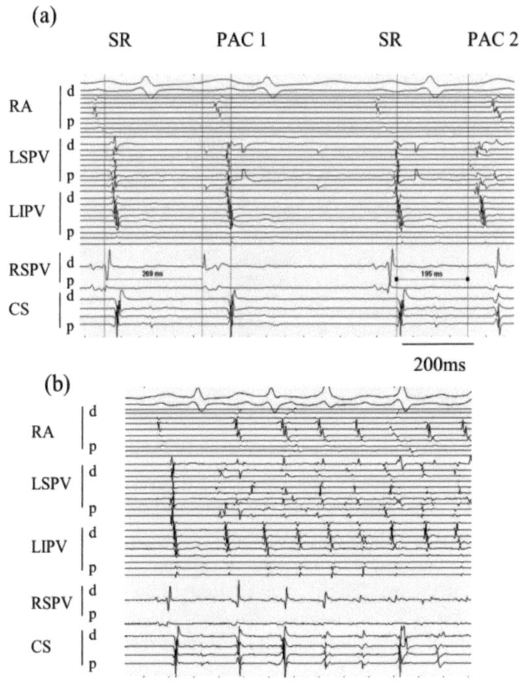

Figure 2. Multiple foci from the right and left PVs. The electrogram exhibiting the PV foci is a two-component electrogram during sinus rhythm. Premature atrial beats one from the right superior PV (a). The electrogram of the ectopic beat exhibits a reversal polarity and a rapid deflection with a coupling interval of 269 ms and apparently precedes the P-wave onset recorded in the 12 ECG. The following PAC 2 originating from the left superior PV spontaneously occurred with a coupling interval of 195 ms. The frequency of PAC 1 and PAC 2 gradually developed, and then PAC 2 was finally shifted to AF (b).

in the superior vena cava (21 %), LA posterior wall (14 %), terminal crest (7.4 %), coronary sinus (7.4 %), left lateral area (6.9 %), LA roof (4.6 %), atrial septum (3.7 %), and other sites (1. 5%). Non-PV foci were detected before the PV isolation procedure in 55 of 109 foci (50 %) (superior vena cava (77 %), atrial septum (39 %), terminal crest (38 %), coronary sinus (38 %), LA roof (24 %), left lateral area (20 %), LA posterior wall (13 %)). The roving catheter had to be relocated to search for the foci uncovered by the catheters in 58 of 214 patients (27 %). PV foci were significantly more related to AF occurrence than non-PV foci (PV foci 61 % vs. non-PV foci 28 %, $p<0.001$]. The mean coupling interval of PV foci was significantly shorter than that of non-PV foci (196±68 vs. 255±90ms, $p<0.001$]. The number of inducible foci was significantly higher in patients with non-PV foci than without those (3.1±1.7 vs. 1.5±1.4, $p<0.001$].

Non-PV foci were induced 15 % of the time with no ISP, 30 % with 1–2 g/min, and 55 % with 2–20 g/min. PV foci were revealed 25 % of the time with no ISP, 43 % with 1–2 g/min, and 32 % with 2–20 g/min. The distribution of the inducibility according to the ISP dose significantly differed between PV foci and non-PV foci ($p<0.001$).

In half of the enrolled patients, non-PV foci were confirmed and accounted for one third of all AMF. High-dose ISP could improve the ratio of the detection of both PV and non-PV foci;

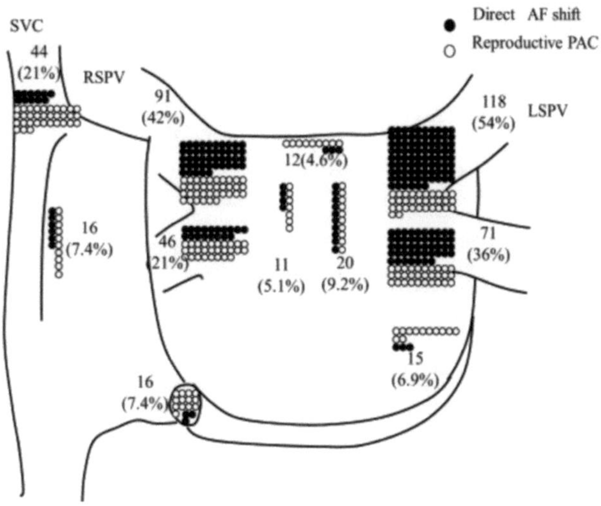

Figure 3. The location of induced AMF. AMF were determined as direct AF triggers or spontaneous reproductive premature atrial premature contraction (PAC) with the coupling interval less than 350 ms or repetitive firing in arrhythmogenic foci. Black circle represents foci which directly shifted to AF; white circle represents reproductive PAC and repetitive firing. To detect the location of foci, we simultaneously used five multipolar catheters to record the electrograms outside the PVs, coronary sinus, SVC, and crista terminalis to search for the AMF during isoproterenol administration.

however, the dose of the ISP was significantly higher for the non-PV foci than the PV foci. The predominant non-PV trigger sites seemed to be related to anatomical structures such as the terminal crest or ligament/vein of Marshall, known to be catecholamine-sensitive structures [5]. These evidences may explain why a high dose of ISP was needed to reveal non-PV foci.

2.3. The PV/non-PV arrhythmogenic foci between paroxysmal and persistent AF

. The incidence of PV foci and non-PV foci from the left atrium was not significantly different between paroxysmal and persistent AF patients. The incidence of non-PV foci, the sum number of foci, the number of non-PV foci, the incidence of right atrial foci, and the occurrence of multiple foci were significantly higher in the persistent than paroxysmal AF. In a multivariate analysis, multiple foci were one of the independent contributing factors to persistent AF as well as the left atrial dimension.

Furthermore, Figure 4 demonstrated that the number of foci was significantly higher in >24 h than < 24 h (1.77±0.16 vs. 2.64±0.14, $p<0.001$) in the paroxysmal AF patients and also significantly higher <1 year than >1 year (3.62±0.15 vs. 1.92±0.16, $p=0.038$) in persistent AF patients. In the data of comparing the AF incidence from PV/non-PV foci between paroxysmal and persistent AF, PV foci were confirmed in 86 % >24 h and in 94 % < 24 h in paroxysmal AF patients and in 96 % <1 year and in 86 % >1 year in persistent AF patients. Non-PV foci were confirmed in 32 % >24 h and in 58 % < 24 h in the paroxysmal AF and in 66 % <1 year and in 59 % >1 year in the persistent AF. The number of foci was significantly increased with a longer AF period in paroxysmal AF, whereas it had significant association on a short AF period in persistent AF. Therefore, these findings may imply that the presence of increased foci may possibly facilitate the development of a shift from paroxysmal to persistent AF, although that may gradually become less significant as long-lasting AF develops.

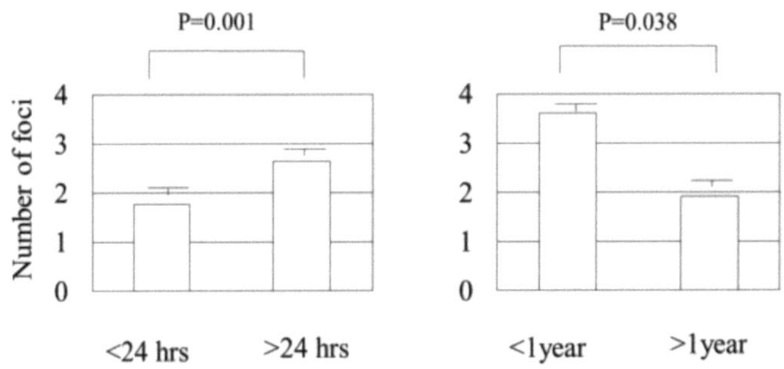

Figure 4. The number of induced foci between paroxysmal and persistent AF. The left graph demonstrates the comparison of the number of foci between those with episodes of < 24 h (n=70) and > 24 h (n=82) in patients with paroxysmal AF. The right graph shows the comparison between AF episodes < 1 year (n=19) and those > 1 year (n=21) in persisted AF patients. The number of foci was significantly higher in >24 h than < 24 h (1.77±0.16 vs. 2.64±0.14, $p<0.001$) in the paroxysmal AF patients and significantly higher <1 year than >1 year (3.62±0.15 vs. 1.92±0.16, p=0.038) in the persistent AF patients. These evidences may imply that the presence of multiple foci may help the promotion from paroxysmal to persistent AF state, and long-lasting AF might reduce the significance of the multiple foci in the perpetuation of AF.

AF occurrence after ablation was significantly higher in patients with multiple foci than without it (sum; 26 % vs. 11 %, p=0.024, paroxysmal; 22 % vs. 14 %, p=0.087, persistent; 26 % vs. 19 %, p=0.630). The hazard ratio of multiple foci being associated with recurrent AF demonstrated that those foci were not a significant relating factor for recurrent AF (2.03 (0.92–3.76), p=0.106).

The multiple triggers may allow a greater chance of reinitiating AF even after the AF self-termination and may facilitate the progression to the persistency from a paroxysmal to persistent AF. In the meantime, the enhanced triggered activity of multiple sites as the cause of AF persistency could also beget AF perpetuation by making new wavelets and less likelihood of AF self-termination. Furthermore, the enhanced dispersion of the atrial refractoriness may also be a crucial factor for AF persistency. The presence of increased atrial dispersion might promote the progression from paroxysmal to persistent AF state [21]. These observations may provide a clue as to why multiple triggers are associated with the development of the fibrillatory process in AF persistency.

2.4. Mutual linkage of left PV AMF

PV myocardial sleeves with complex muscle bundle orientations or specific autonomic nervous system may have the same interactions between each PV. Thus, we determined the mutual linkage of AMF around PVs. AFC from the left superior PV were significantly associated with AFC of the left inferior PV (42 % vs. 23 %, $p<0.05$), left-sided left posterior wall (20 % vs. 5 %, $p<0.05$), and roof area (8 % vs. 2 %, $p<0.05$) (Figure 5). In case of foci from LSPV, the occurrence of AMF was 68 % in LIPV, 85 % in the left side LA posterior wall, and 75 % in the roof. Right PVs had no significant mutual association for AFC between each other (Figure 6).

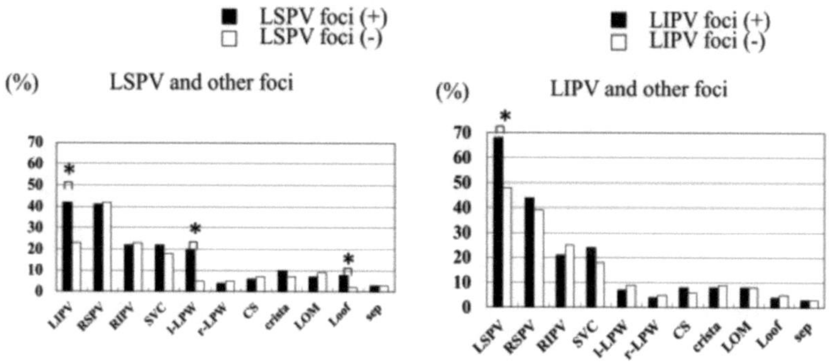

Figure 5. The relation between left PV foci and other foci. The incidence of foci from LIPV (42 % vs. 23, p<0.05), left-side left atrial posterior wall (20 % vs. 5 %, p<0.05) and left atrial roof (8 % vs. 2 %, p<0.05) was highly detected in patients with LSPV than without LSPV foci.

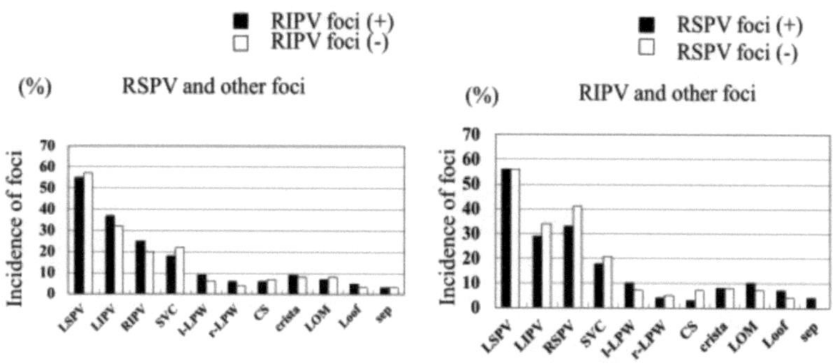

Figure 6. The relation between right PV foci and other foci. There is no significant relation between right PV foci and other foci.

Left lateral ridge as the anterior wall of left PVs facilitating to connect both superior and inferior PV may contribute the mutual arrhythmogenic linkage of them. Thus, we examined the relation between the shape of left lateral ridge and LPV's arrhythmogenicity in 120 AF patients.

Morphology of the left lateral ridge was determined by the endoscopic view of 64-MDCT. From the relation to superior and inferior PVs, the characteristics of the ridge was classified into 3 groups: long (connecting both PVs, n=44), intermediate (half of PV distance, n=53), and poor (only around PV, n=23) (Figure 7). The incidence of AF foci from the left inferior PV (29 % vs. 9 %, p<0.05) and spontaneous AF occurrence from both PVs (23 % vs. 5 %, p<0.05) were significantly higher in the long type than in the intermediate and short types. The number of AF foci around the ridge was significantly greater in patients with long type than those without it (1.2±0.9 vs. 0.6±0.7, p<0.01).

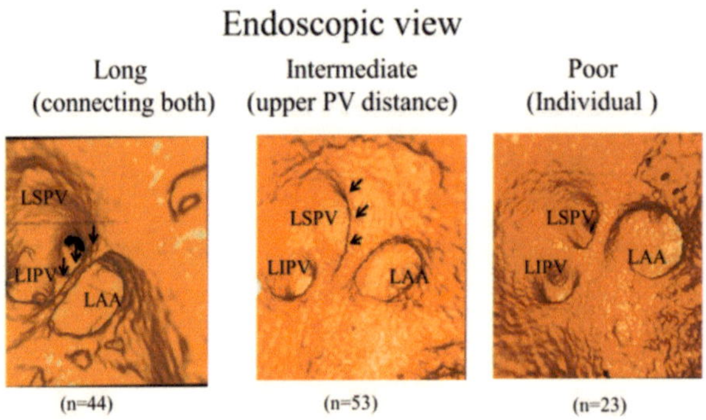

Figure 7. Endoscopic view of left PVs ostium. LSPV, left superior pulmonary vein; LIPV, left inferior pulmonary vein; LAA, left atrial appendage.

2.5. Left atrial roof shape and PV/non-PV foci

The remodeling process is associated with the structural and electrophysiological abnormality in the PVs and atrium, which could promote local conduction delay and lead to an increased PV/non-PV arrhythmogenicity developing to AF persistency [15, 16, 17, 10, 11]. These evidences might imply that the morphological features of the PVs and atrium can contain a crucial role to detect their preexisting arrhythmogenicity, although the evaluation of the morphological features is limited in a quantitative manner because of their variable and unique structure.

The left atrial (LA) roof consisting of the upper wall of the left atrium and upper PVs was demonstrated as the silhouette of LA roof and could simply be visualized by PV angiography or left atrial CT imaging. In addition, the dominancy of morphological PVs/LA and the features of the LA roof silhouette could be easily determined in patients with AF. Thus, the relation between PV/non-PV arrhythmogenicity and LA roof silhouette was examined in this study.

Based on the PVs and LA dominancy, The LA roof shape was classified into a deep V shape (possible PV dominancy), shallow V shape, and flat-coved shape (possible LA dominancy) by cine angiography (Figure 8]. Angiography was conducted by both contrast media from the long sheath locating at the right and left superior PVs. The LA roof shape was assessed by A–P projection and was determined by the angle of the LA roof silhouette between the right and left LA wall. The deep V shape was defined as <140°, shallow V shape was 140° to180°, and flat-coved shape was > 180°.

Table 2 shows the relation between AMF and roof-shape group. In results, 335 AMF were detected. PV/ non-PV foci were observed in 136 of 152 (89 %) AF patients. AF triggers immediately shifting to AF were found in 114/152 (75 %) AF patients, and AF from PV foci was in 84 of 152 (55 %) AF patients. PV foci containing reproducible atrial premature contractions were observed in 135 of 152 AF patients (89 %) and non-PV foci in 77 of 152 (44 %). The location of non-PV foci was in the superior vena cava (25, 28 %), left atrial posterior wall (19, 21 %), terminal crest (10, 11 %), CS (10, 11 %), left lateral area (9, 10 %), LA roof (7, 8 %), atrial septum (4, 4 %), and other areas (6, 7 %).

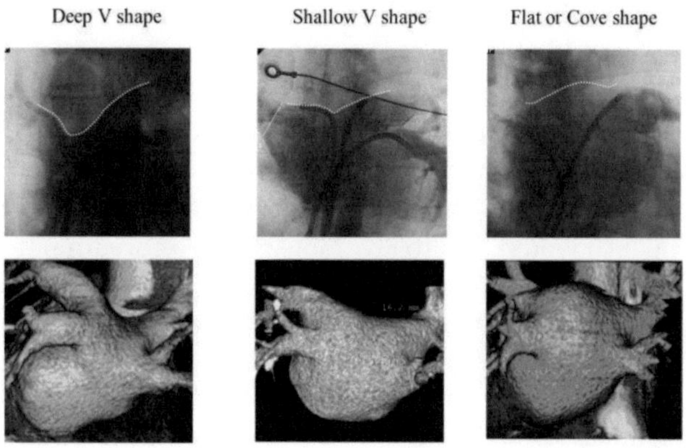

Figure 8. According to the PV and LA dominant level, the LA roof shapes into a deep V shape, shallow V shape, and flat-coved shape which were classified by using cineangiography and 64-slice MDCT. The upper figure is the cineangiography, and the lower is the 3D-constructed image of the MDCT. The deep V shape seemed to be dominated by the segment of both trunks of the upper PVs, whereas the flat-coved LA roof shape shows less incorporation into the LA.

As the silhouette of LA roof got to flat, the incidence of AF from the PVs (deep V 70 % vs. shallow V 57 % vs. flat 40 %, p=0.003), AF of the upper PVs (deep V 63 % vs. shallow V 41 % vs. flat 38 %, p=0.046), and PV foci including reproducible premature contractions (deep V 94 % vs. shallow V 84 % vs. flat 76 %, p=0.033) significantly decreased. The incidence of AF from non-PV sites (sharp V 6 % vs. shallow V 13 % vs. flat 22 %, p=0.041) and non-PV foci including atrial premature contractions (sharp V 26 % vs. shallow V 46 % vs. flat 54 %, p=0.016) were significantly increased as the LA roof silhouette got to flat. In a multivariate analysis, the deep V was an independent relating factor to PV AF triggers (OR 2.94 (1.27–6.80), p=0.012). These findings may include the novelty of the LA roof silhouette as an index of the PV's arrhythmogenicity.

AF is likely to originate from larger PVs [22], and the enlarged PVs may often be associated with the arrhythmogenic PVs [23]. Enlarged PV by the atrial stretch can enhance the PV's automaticity and triggered activity for AF initiation [24]. In addition, the atrial remodeling process may promote the increased triggered activity of non-PV lesions. The presence of multiple PV/non-PV foci could be related to longer AF duration, an older age, and larger atrial dimensions [25]. And also, LA enlargement could predispose LA posterior wall triggers [15].

3. Marshall bundle and arrhythmogenic foci

Marshall reported that a "vestigial fold of the pericardium" lies dorsal to the left atrial appendage in 1850. The small oblique vein of Marshall (VOM) is often connected to the vestigial folds going around the ostium of the left PVs. VOM drains into CS and separates the great cardiac vein and CS. The muscle sleeves of the VOM are also connected to CS musculature [26]. The vein or its ligament of Marshall is usually connected to the left PVs [27, 28, 29], and its distal ends are directly connected to the posterior wall of the left atrium [27, 30].

AF can originate from VOM or its ligament because of its catecholamine-sensitive structure [31, 5]. Preserved persistent left superior vena cava as a remnant of VOM can also include the similar electrical and anatomical features [32]. VOM or its ligament has connections to muscle bundles of the left atrium as well as of the surrounding coronary sinus (CS) in histological studies. The distal end often connects to the LA lateral area and to the left PVs [27, 29]. Therefore, recognition of the VOM anatomy in AF patients would help access to non-PV foci around the left PVs, which would lead to favorable clinical procedural result.

3.1. Angiographic vein of Marshall and AMF

In 100 AF patients, we examined the anatomy of VOM with balloon-occluded venography of coronary sinus using a balloon wedge pressure catheter (Goodtec, Huntington Beach, CA). The landmark of VOM orifice was identified at the junction of the CS and great cardiac vein. The right anterior oblique, left anterior oblique, and anteroposterior views were obtained in enrolled AF patients (Figure 9). To identify the anatomical association for VOM to both the superior and inferior left PVs, we performed selective superior and left inferior left PVs angiography by using injection of 5–10 ml of contrast medium from long sheaths. The grade of VOM development was measured from the AP view and classified into two grades (poor, reaching below superior left PV distributed in LA, and good, above superior left PVs).

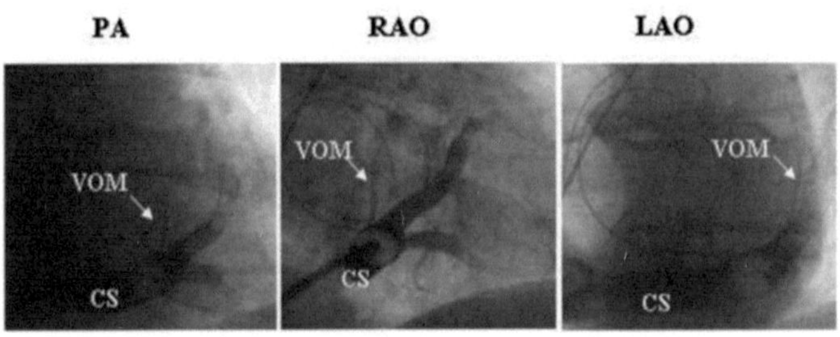

Figure 9. Representative results of VOM angiography. The location of the VOM is indicated by arrows. VOM runs obliquely between the left atrial appendage and LSPV.

VOM was visualized by balloon-occluded CS venography in 73 AF patients (73 %). There were no significant differences in clinical characteristics of the two groups. VOM development was poor in 55 patients (75 %) and good in 18 patients. In the anteroposterior image, the VOM running behind the mitral isthmus line was confirmed. VOM going through the mitral isthmus area was observed in 51 patients (51 %). The branches originating from the end of VOM was observed in 49 patients (67 %).

The incidence of PV foci from the left superior PV was significantly higher in patients with VOM than in those without it (66 % vs. 42 %, P=0. 05). And also, the incidence of left superior PV foci as direct AF initiator was significantly higher in patients with VOM than in those without it (50 % vs. 30 %, P<0. 05). The incidences of e left superior PV foci were 41 % in none, 69 % in poor VOM, and 56 % in good VOM. The incidences of the left superior PV foci as direct AF initiator were 30 % in none, 56 % in poor VOM, and 33 % in good VOM.

http://dx.doi.org/10.5772/60646

Twelve patients had non-PV foci in the LA posterior wall, and nine (75 %) of these patients also had PV foci in the left superior PV around VOM structure even after the successful PV isolation procedure at PV ostium level. The correlation between angiographic VOM anatomy and surrounding non-PV foci is shown in Figure 4. After ablating the site at the branch of VOM connecting to the LA wall, we can often successfully terminate AF. Twenty-eight patients had 30 non-PV foci surrounding left superior PVs including LA posterior free wall, LA roof, and LA lateral wall, and 12 of 30 non-PV foci were directly shifted to AF.

The branches of the VOM were a good landmark to identify the location of non-PV foci around left PVs (Figure 10). We could successfully ablate the residual non-PV foci at the distal end of VOM in 11 patients (39 %) after PV ostial isolation (AF termination after RF delivery, 3; disappearance of reproductive atrial premature contractions, 8). Successful terminations of non-PV foci were observed in 5 in left LA posterior wall, 4 in LA lateral wall, and 2 in LA roof. Among 28 patients with non-PV foci surrounding left PVs, non-PV foci were successfully deleted in 17 patients, whereas 11 patients of them had AF recurrence. Seven of 11 (67 %) with successful non-PV foci termination were free from AF recurrence.

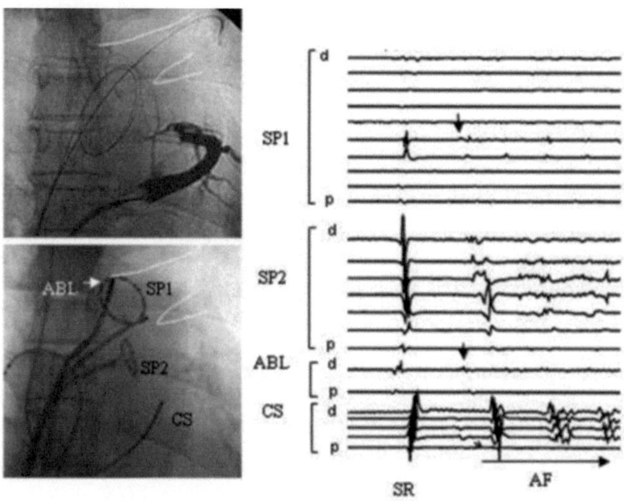

Figure 10. Spontaneous PV and coronary sinus angiography (3a). The VOM reached between LSPV and LIPV and ran laterally to the LIPV ostium. Super-selective VOM angiography revealed that the end of VOM had a branch that spreads in the area of the lateral and posterior wall below the LSPV ostium (3b). Arrows indicate the end of the VOM.

The presence of VOM is associated with a higher incidence of AF triggers of the left superior PVs. The incidence of left superior PV foci was significantly higher in patients with visible VOM than in those without visible VOM. In angiographic findings, the distal braches of VOM are commonly distributed around both the left superior and inferior PVs, especially in patients with good visual VOM. The VOM and its ligament richly innervated by sympathetic nerves could be served as a cause of isoproterenol-sensitive automatic activity [5, 33]. These evidences support arrhythmogenic foci from the VOM, and its ligament can be inducible by using high-dose isoproterenol administration.

Left PVs foci and non-PV foci adjacent to the left PVs can have an influence on each other. Approximately 40 % of non-PV foci around the left superior PV were successfully ablated by targeting the distal end of VOM or its branches. These evidences demonstrate the angiographic data of VOM, and its branches may indicate the site of catheter ablation of non-PV foci. Radiofrequency energy applied to the areas of VOM distal ends occasionally delineated non-PV foci originating from the surrounding area of left PVs. Thus, we believe that understanding of the VOM anatomy can improve the clinical outcome of ablation in cases with catecholamine-sensitive AF.

3.2. Conduction along the left lateral ridge and the arrhythmogenicity of the left pulmonary veins

The ligament and VOM containing the Marshall bundle (MB) with richly innervates the sympathetic and parasympathetic nerves is within the left lateral ridge (LLR) which is longitudinally running between the left atrial appendage and left pulmonary vein (LPVs), and they can serve as a source of triggers and the substrate of reentry of atrial fibrillation (AF) [1,2]. If the distinctive dominant conduction along the LLR is present, possibly due to the continuous and/or partial MB conduction, its conduction may be associated with the increased arrhythmogenicity of the LPVs. In this study, we examined the relationship between the preferential conduction properties of the MB and the arrhythmogenicity of the LPVs in 40 AF patients.

A 20-pole diagnostic catheter was positioned in the CS for pacing and recording. The upper and lower LPVs were simultaneously mapped with two adjustable 20-pole catheters (Optima, Irvine, USA) (Figure 11a). At first, RF energy during CS pacing was delivered along the LLR as a part of the LPV ablation (Figure 11b), and each ablation site and the conduction pattern during the RF delivery were monitored and recorded by fluoroscopy and a 3D electroanatomical system.

The earliest activated site of the upper LPV during CS pacing was observed at the carina lesion in 32 of 40 patients (80 %), anterior wall in four of 40 (10 %), and posterior wall in four of 40 (10 %). The earliest activated site was at the upper LPV in 34 of 40 (85 %), bottom of the lower LPV in four of 40 (10 %), and posterior site in two of 40 (5 %).

After the RF delivery along the LLR, the PV potentials of the upper LPV completely disappeared in one patient and that of the lower LPV in two patients. The conduction time between the LPVs and CS stimulus site was significantly prolonged during the RF delivery (before vs. after; upper, 91±26 ms vs. 127±38 ms, $p<0.001$; lower, 86±21ms vs. 103±22ms, $p<0.001$). A remarkable prolongation of more than 30 ms was observed in 19 of 40 patients (48 %) (both LPVs, 6; only the upper LPVs, 12; and only the lower LPV, 1). The sites of the remarkable prolongation during the RF delivery were observed at the carina between the LPVs [4], anterior site of the upper LPV carina [10], anterior wall of the lower LPV [3], and bottom of the lower LPVs [2].

Thirty-three AMF from LPVs (upper, 22; lower, 11) were observed in 23/40 patients (56 %). Fifteen of the detected foci directly shifted to AF, and 16 of them exhibited premature atrial contractions and/or transient frequent repetitive firings. The earliest activated site of the AMF

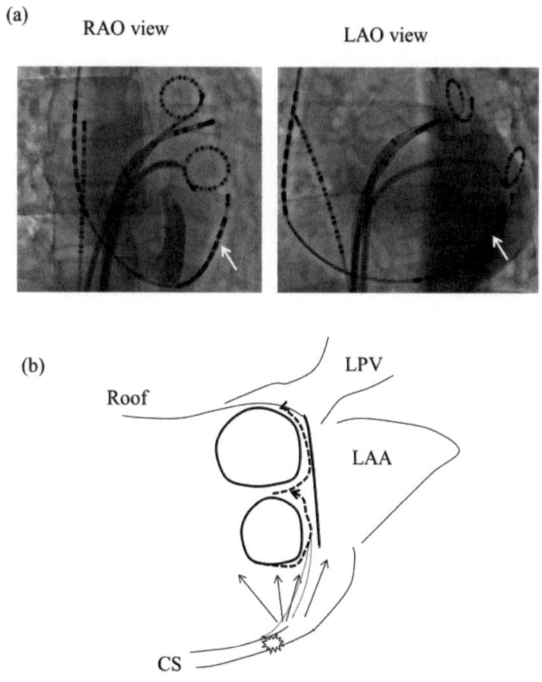

Figure 11. The location of the PV/non-PV foci showing the earliest atrial focus was determined by a reference for the local electrogram and the earliest activation site of the foci. The earliest activation sites from arrhythmogenic foci and during CS pacing were determined by the direction of the spontaneous activation recorded by double spiral catheters located in both LPVs. The pacing site during the RF application was delivered from the posterolateral CS, possibly from the takeoff site of the MB. The RF application along the LLR was sequentially delivered in a lower to upper manner (from the bottom of the inferior LPV, anterior wall of the inferior LPV, and LPV carina to the anterior wall of the superior LPV) during CS pacing.

from the upper LPV was found at the carina region in 12 of 22 (55 %), anterior wall in three of 22 (14 %), roof site in three of 22 (14 %), and posterior wall in four of 22 (18 %). The earliest activated site of the AMF from the lower LPV was found at the carina region in six of 11 (55 %), anterior wall in two of 11 (18 %), bottom in one of 11 (9 %), and posterior wall in two of 11 (18 %).

The conduction time from the CS to the earliest activated upper PV after the RF delivery was significantly longer in patients with AMF from the upper LPV than in those patients without (107±36 ms vs. 146±40 ms, $p<0.01$), and the conduction time from the CS pacing site to the earliest activation site of the upper LPV was significantly prolonged in the patients with AMF than in those without during the RF delivery (44±22ms vs. 17±11ms, $p<0.01$).

In this study, the earliest site of AMF from the LPVs was often determined to be around the carina region. These observations are likely to be consistent with the previous report [9]. In addition, the complex crossing of the muscular connections, bridges, neural inputs, and the adjoining muscle sleeves, possibly related to the MB conduction in the inter-PV carina, might promote electrical arrhythmogenicity including spontaneous ectopies of AF [10]. And also, the earliest activated site of the upper LPVs during CS pacing was highly observed around the carina region, and also a remarkable prolongation jump during the RF delivery was highly observed around the carina and/or adjacent anterior area. A previous report suggested that the distal exit of the MB into the upper LPV is commonly located around the inter-PV junction, possibly bypassing the LPV junction to the left atrium [34]. These specific muscle orientations and the dominant MB conduction toward the carina region could promote the preferential conduction properties.

In addition, the prolongation of the conduction time between the CS and LPVs during the RF delivery was significantly more commonly observed in patients with upper LPV AMF than in those without. The preferential properties of the MB connecting to the LPVs might involve cross talk that promotes an increased LPV arrhythmogenicity [3, 4, 11]. A larger amount of preserved MB muscle as a remnant of the LSVC, which is related to the conduction properties of the LPVs, may be crucial for determining the increased arrhythmogenicity of the LPVs.

4. The efficacy of the sinus restoration strategy to detect arrhythmogenic foci for persistent AF

Catheter ablation (CA) of persistent AF may commonly be performed during ongoing AF, mainly targeting sites exhibiting complex atrial fractionated electrograms (CFAEs) and/or dominant frequencies (DFs) in addition to pulmonary vein (PV) isolation [35, 36, 37]. However, CA during ongoing AF may be limited especially in patients with a trigger dominant-type AF [20,38, 19]. The rapid firing from the PVs and non-PV foci may beget enhanced automaticity, triggered activity, and localized micro-reentry as AF initiation and maintenance [37, 3, 10].

Our prior data suggested that an increased number of AMF are more highly observed during a vigorous sinus rhythm (SR) restoration strategy in persistent rather than paroxysmal AF [39], and the failure of the elimination of the AMF initiating an immediate recurrence of AF was significantly associated with the recurrence of persistent AF [40]. In this study, we performed CA based on a vigorous SR restoration strategy for persistent AF and evaluated the relationship between the electrophysiological features of the inducible AMF and recurrent AF episodes after the CA in 117 persistent AF patients.

The AF ablation strategy is summarized in Figure 12. We initially performed the PV isolation procedure by using a double circular mapping catheter technique. The DC energy was delivered with an external biphasic waveform of up to 270 J before the PV isolation. The electrical PV isolation was successfully accomplished with monitoring the circumferential electrical isolation at the antrum level: approximately 1–2 cm from of both the right and left PVs ostium.

After the PV isolation procedure, an additional RF energy application was primarily applied to create an LA roof line. When the AF was still persisted or inducible after LA roof line, additional mitral isthmus line or ablation of the area showing complex fractionated atrial electrograms (CFAEs) in left atrium was accomplished. When AF could not be terminated in

http://dx.doi.org/10.5772/60646

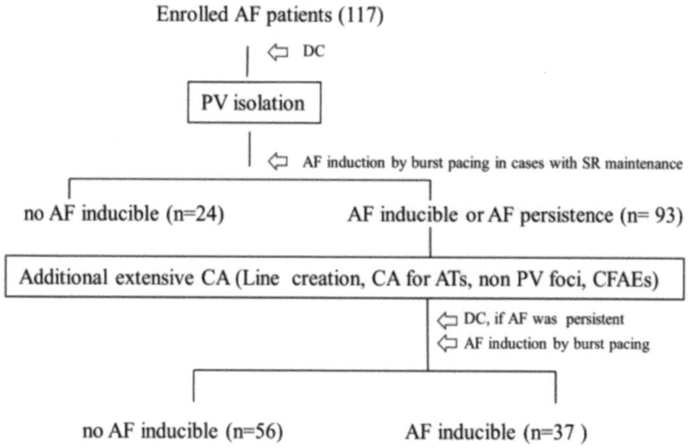

Figure 12. The summarized vigorous SR restoration strategy during the ablation according to the pacing-oriented AF inducibility. SR rhythm was restored by using external direct cardioversion before the PV isolation and line creation at the end of the ablation. AF was no longer inducible after only the PV isolation procedure in 24 of 117 patients (20.5 %). During the PV isolation, SR shifted to AF spontaneously and/or was triggered by the roving catheter in 68 of 117 patients

these series of procedures, direct cardioversion was delivered to restore SR again in such cases. Then, we confirmed whether complete block lines were created at the roof and mitral isthmus.

Extensive electrical isolation for PVs was successfully performed in all enrolled patients. An LA roof line was additionally created in 93 of 117 (80 %) patients after the extensive PV delineation, and the successful block line was confirmed in 86 of 93 patients (92 %). ATs were inducible in 61 of 117 patients (52.1 %) during the CA (tricuspid-dependent AT, 30; mitral annulus-dependent AT, 15; septal through, 5; LA anterior, 5; and upper loop in right atrium, 3). ATs with an unstable circuit were observed in five patients. A mitral isthmus line was additionally created in 34 of 117 patients (29 %). We confirmed a successful mitral block in 22 of 34 patients (65 %). Epicardial approach from the CS was needed in 18 out of 34 patients (53 %). Ablation targeted to the CFAEs was performed in 19 of 117 patients (16 %). Three common atrioventricular nodal reentry tachycardias (AVNRT) and one sinus nodal tachycardia (SANRT) were induced and successfully terminated.

At the end of the CA, residual AF could still be induced in 37 out of 117 patients (31.6 %), and also residual ATs were still inducible in 30 of 117 (25.6 %) (MI-dependent AT, 5; localized in LA anterior, 3; LA septal, 1; stable unknown, 11; and unstable, 11). Cardiac tamponade occurred in one of 117 (0.85 %) patients during the ablation. A nonsurgical drainage was successfully performed in those cases. The mean procedural time was 174±35 min, and the mean fluoroscopic time was 52±16.8 min.

At the end of the CA, residual AMF were still found in 48 of 117 patients (41.0 %) (directly shifted to AF, 22; reproducible atrial premature beats, [26]. The locations included the left atrial posterior wall [6], superior vena cava [3], crista terminalis [4], left lateral area [1], interatrial septum [1], coronary sinus ostium [1], and unknown [32]. The number of AMF during the CA was significantly higher in the patients with residual AMF than in those without (2.3±1.2 vs. 3.0±1.2, p=0.041).

The incidence of non-PV AMF was significantly higher in the patients with pacing inducible AF than in those without [69 % vs. 47 %, p=0.032). The residual AMF were significantly higher in the patients with pacing-inducible AF than in those without (67 % vs. 29 %, p<0.001).

The mean follow-up period after the CA was 937 days. The follow-up ratio was 106 out of 117 patients (90.6 %) at one year and 86 of 117 patients (73.5 %) at two years after the CA. In-hospital AF episodes were observed in 17 of 117 (14.5 %) patients, and a long-term AF recurrence was observed in 42 of 117 (35.9 %) patients. AT episodes after the CA were observed in 31 of 117 patients (26.4 %), and those were only observed within 3 months after the CA in 11 of 31 patients (35.4 %). AT episodes coexisted with the AF episodes in 16 of 31 patients (52 %). In the multivariable analysis, the AF duration (1.01 (1.00–1.02), p=0.012), LA volume (1.01 (1.01–1.02), p=0.006), and residual AMF (3.95 (1.32–11.8), p=0.004) were independent risk factors for recurrent AF. Figure 13 demonstrates the AF recurrence ratio in the patients with and without residual AMF. AF episodes after the CA were significantly greater in the patients with residual AMF than in those without (50 % vs. 26 %, p=0.002). The result of the study demonstrated that the residual AMF was a useful predicting parameter for the outcome of CA, and the clinical course was impressively favorable in patients without residual AMF (AF recurrence after initial session at two years was 26%). (58.1 %). At the end of the ablation, residual AF was still inducible in 37 of 117 patients (31.6 %).

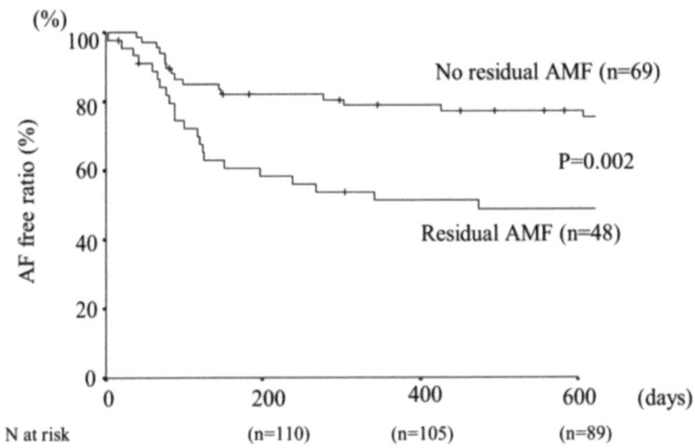

Figure 13. The AF recurrence ratio in the patients with and without residual arrhythmogenic foci during the follow-up. Residual foci were observed in 48 of 117 patients (41 %). The AF free ratio between both groups was compared by a log rank analysis, and AF episodes after the CA were significantly higher in the patients with residual foci than in those without (50 % vs. 26 %, p=0.002). The mean follow-up period was 937 days.

After only a PV isolation, AF was no longer inducible in approximately one fifth of the patients with a favorable outcome even though they underwent a less aggressive intervention. This information might allow us to reduce the number of unnecessary additional RF applications during CA. On the other hand, non-PV foci were also highly confirmed even in patients with persistent AF [39]. Several studies have also addressed the importance of modifying the non-PV foci to improve the outcome of CA for AF [20, 23]. A vigorous SR restoration strategy might facilitate determining the non-PV arrhythmogenicity.

The data from this study also showed that non-PV AMF were closely associated with the AF pacing inducibility during CA. The development of the atrial remodeling process might enhance the triggered activity of the non-PV lesions, because the increased non-PV arrhythmogenicity may be associated with the atrial remodeling process including an enlarged LA [25, 41]. A recent study demonstrated that the response to ISP after CA more accurately predicted AF recurrences in patients with paroxysmal AF [38]. Residual AMF could increase the chance of AF initiation, and the significance of those may be especially pronounced particularly in cases that develop atrial remodeling.

In conclusion, these data support the role of arrhythmic triggers in determining eventual recurrences in patients with persistent AF and point to AMF as a potentially valuable early index of long-term ablation success.

5. Conclusions

AMF could be involved in mechanism of the AF development. In addition, atrial anatomical structure such as left atrial roof shape, left lateral ridge, and Marshall vein provided us with an understanding of the arrhythmogenicity of the PVs and non-PVs in patients with AF. Because the presence of residual AMF is associated with increased AF recurrence after ablation, the information of AMF is useful for determining the appropriate strategy of ablation for AF.

Author details

Toshiya Kurotobi*

Address all correspondence to: drk21cent@gmail.com

Shiroyama Hospital, Division of Cardiac Rhythm Management, Japan

References

[1] Haissaguerre M, Jais P, Shah DC et al. Spontaneous initiation of atrial fibrillation by ectopic beats originating in the pulmonary veins. N Engl J Med 1998;339:659-66.

[2] Chugh A, Oral H, Lemola K et al. Prevalence, mechanisms, and clinical significance of macroreentrant atrial tachycardia during and following left atrial ablation for atrial fibrillation. Heart Rhythm 2005;2:464-71.

[3] Patterson E, Lazzara R, Szabo B et al. Sodium-calcium exchange initiated by the Ca2+ transient: an arrhythmia trigger within pulmonary veins. J Am Coll Cardiol 2006;47:1196-206.

[4] Cherry EM, Ehrlich JR, Nattel S, Fenton FH. Pulmonary vein reentry--properties and size matter: insights from a computational analysis. Heart Rhythm 2007;4:1553-62.

[5] Hwang C, Wu TJ, Doshi RN, Peter CT, Chen PS. Vein of marshall cannulation for the analysis of electrical activity in patients with focal atrial fibrillation. Circulation 2000;101:1503-5.

[6] Chen SA, Tai CT, Yu WC et al. Right atrial focal atrial fibrillation: electrophysiologic characteristics and radiofrequency catheter ablation. J Cardiovasc Electrophysiol 1999;10:328-35.

[7] Cappato R, Negroni S, Pecora D et al. Prospective assessment of late conduction recurrence across radiofrequency lesions producing electrical disconnection at the pulmonary vein ostium in patients with atrial fibrillation. Circulation 2003;108:1599-604.

[8] Mangrum JM, Mounsey JP, Kok LC, DiMarco JP, Haines DE. Intracardiac echocardiography-guided, anatomically based radiofrequency ablation of focal atrial fibrillation originating from pulmonary veins. J Am Coll Cardiol 2002;39:1964-72.

[9] Schmitt C, Ndrepepa G, Weber S et al. Biatrial multisite mapping of atrial premature complexes triggering onset of atrial fibrillation. Am J Cardiol 2002;89:1381-7.

[10] Chen YJ, Chen YC, Yeh HI, Lin CI, Chen SA. Electrophysiology and arrhythmogenic activity of single cardiomyocytes from canine superior vena cava. Circulation 2002;105:2679-85.

[11] Johnson N, Danilo P, Jr., Wit AL, Rosen MR. Characteristics of initiation and termination of catecholamine-induced triggered activity in atrial fibers of the coronary sinus. Circulation 1986;74:1168-79.

[12] Scherlag BJ, Yeh BK, Robinson MJ. Inferior interatrial pathway in the dog. Circ Res 1972;31:18-35.

[13] Wit AL, Cranefield PF. Triggered activity in cardiac muscle fibers of the simian mitral valve. Circ Res 1976;38:85-98.

[14] Saito T, Otoguro M, Matsubara T. Electrophysiological studies on the mechanism of electrically induced sustained rhythmic activity in the rabbit right atrium. Circ Res 1978;42:199-206.

[15] Lee SH, Tai CT, Hsieh MH et al. Predictors of non-pulmonary vein ectopic beats initiating paroxysmal atrial fibrillation: implication for catheter ablation. J Am Coll Cardiol 2005;46:1054-9.

[16] Wijffels MC, Kirchhof CJ, Dorland R, Allessie MA. Atrial fibrillation begets atrial fibrillation. A study in awake chronically instrumented goats. Circulation 1995;92:1954-68.

[17] Hoit BD, Shao Y, Gabel M. Left atrial systolic and diastolic function accompanying chronic rapid pacing-induced atrial failure. Am J Physiol 1998;275:H183-9.

[18] Arora R, Verheule S, Scott L et al. Arrhythmogenic substrate of the pulmonary veins assessed by high-resolution optical mapping. Circulation 2003;107:1816-21.

[19] Kurotobi T, Ito H, Inoue K et al. Marshall vein as arrhythmogenic source in patients with atrial fibrillation: correlation between its anatomy and electrophysiological findings. J Cardiovasc Electrophysiol 2006;17:1062-7.

[20] Lin WS, Tai CT, Hsieh MH et al. Catheter ablation of paroxysmal atrial fibrillation initiated by non-pulmonary vein ectopy. Circulation 2003;107:3176-83.

[21] Koide Y, Yotsukura M, Ando H et al. Usefulness of P-wave dispersion in standard twelve-lead electrocardiography to predict transition from paroxysmal to persistent atrial fibrillation. Am J Cardiol 2008;102:573-7.

[22] Yamane T, Shah DC, Jais P et al. Dilatation as a marker of pulmonary veins initiating atrial fibrillation. J Interv Card Electrophysiol 2002;6:245-9.

[23] Chen SA, Tai CT, Hsieh MH et al. Radiofrequency catheter ablation of atrial fibrillation initiated by spontaneous ectopic beats. Curr Cardiol Rep 2000;2:322-8.

[24] Satoh T, Zipes DP. Unequal atrial stretch in dogs increases dispersion of refractoriness conducive to developing atrial fibrillation. J Cardiovasc Electrophysiol 1996;7:833-42.

[25] Haissaguerre M, Jais P, Shah DC et al. Electrophysiological end point for catheter ablation of atrial fibrillation initiated from multiple pulmonary venous foci. Circulation 2000;101:1409-17.

[26] Chauvin M, Shah DC, Haissaguerre M, Marcellin L, Brechenmacher C. The anatomic basis of connections between the coronary sinus musculature and the left atrium in humans. Circulation 2000;101:647-52.

[27] Kim DT, Lai AC, Hwang C et al. The ligament of Marshall: a structural analysis in human hearts with implications for atrial arrhythmias. J Am Coll Cardiol 2000;36:1324-7.

[28] Katritsis D, Giazitzoglou E, Korovesis S, Paxinos G, Anagnostopoulos CE, Camm AJ. Epicardial foci of atrial arrhythmias apparently originating in the left pulmonary veins. J Cardiovasc Electrophysiol 2002;13:319-23.

[29] Tan AY, Chou CC, Zhou S et al. Electrical connections between the left superior pulmonary vein, left atrium and ligament of marshall: implications for the mechanisms of atrial fibrillation. Am J Physiol Heart Circ Physiol 2005.

[30] Omichi C, Chou CC, Lee MH et al. Demonstration of electrical and anatomic connections between Marshall bundles and left atrium in dogs: implications on the generation of P waves on surface electrocardiogram. J Cardiovasc Electrophysiol 2002;13:1283-91.

[31] Hwang C, Karagueuzian HS, Chen PS. Idiopathic paroxysmal atrial fibrillation induced by a focal discharge mechanism in the left superior pulmonary vein: possible roles of the ligament of Marshall. J Cardiovasc Electrophysiol 1999;10:636-48.

[32] Haissaguerre M, Sanders P, Hocini M et al. Changes in atrial fibrillation cycle length and inducibility during catheter ablation and their relation to outcome. Circulation 2004;109:3007-13.

[33] Doshi RN, Wu TJ, Yashima M et al. Relation between ligament of Marshall and adrenergic atrial tachyarrhythmia. Circulation 1999;100:876-83.

[34] Hamabe A, Chang CM, Zhou S et al. Induction of atrial fibrillation and nerve sprouting by prolonged left atrial pacing in dogs. Pacing Clin Electrophysiol 2003;26:2247-52.

[35] O'Neill MD, Wright M, Knecht S et al. Long-term follow-up of persistent atrial fibrillation ablation using termination as a procedural endpoint. Eur Heart J 2009;30:1105-12.

[36] Nademanee K. Trials and travails of electrogram-guided ablation of chronic atrial fibrillation. Circulation 2007;115:2592-4.

[37] Lin YJ, Tai CT, Kao T et al. Frequency analysis in different types of paroxysmal atrial fibrillation. J Am Coll Cardiol 2006;47:1401-7.

[38] Crawford T, Chugh A, Good E et al. Clinical value of noninducibility by high-dose isoproterenol versus rapid atrial pacing after catheter ablation of paroxysmal atrial fibrillation. J Cardiovasc Electrophysiol 2010;21:13-20.

[39] Kurotobi T, Iwakura K, Inoue K et al. Multiple AMF associated with the development of perpetuation of atrial fibrillation. Circulation Arrhythmia and Electrophysiology 2010;3:39-45.

[40] Inoue K, Kurotobi T, Kimura R et al. Trigger-based mechanism of the persistence of atrial fibrillation and its impact on the efficacy of catheter ablation. Circulation Arrhythmia and Electrophysiology 2012;5:295-301.

[41] Pak HN, Hwang C, Lim HE, Kim JW, Lee HS, Kim YH. Electroanatomic characteristics of atrial premature beats triggering atrial fibrillation in patients with persistent versus paroxysmal atrial fibrillation. J Cardiovasc Electrophysiol 2006;17:818-24.

Chapter 4

Tachycardia-Induced Cardiomyopathy

Lucie Riedlbauchova

Additional information is available at the end of the chapter

http://dx.doi.org/10.5772/60716

Abstract

Virtually, any kind of tachycardia may lead to the development of tachycardia-induced cardiomyopathy. This term refers to left ventricular dysfunction and dilated cardiomyopathy pattern that occur as a consequence of persistent tachycardia. Impaired left ventricular function in the presence of tachycardia can be found accidentally, but it is often associated with progressive symptoms and signs of heart failure that force the individual to seek medical help. A hallmark of tachycardia-induced cardiomyopathy is the reversibility of both hemodynamic and structural changes after cessation of the index tachycardia. However, contractile dysfunction and structural changes may persist even weeks after the rhythm/rate correction. Therefore, tachycardia-induced cardiomyopathy should be considered as a probable reason of ventricular dysfunction and dilatation in any patient presenting with dilated cardiomyopathy pattern, despite that the initial rhythm is not pathological or the heart rate is well controlled. This review summarizes our current knowledge about this specific form of cardiomyopathy.

Keywords: tachycardia-induced cardiomyopathy, arrhythmia, tachycardia, heart failure, dilated cardiomyopathy

1. Introduction

Cardiomyopathies represent a heterogenous group of myocardial diseases in which the myocardium exhibits structural and/or functional dysfunction [1, 2]. Current definition of cardiomyopathies excludes structural myocardial processes and dysfunction secondary to specific cardiovascular disorders such as coronary artery disease, systemic arterial hypertension, congenital heart diseases or valvular diseases. Although tachycardia-induced cardiomyopathy may be seen as secondary due to well-defined causal cardiovascular factor, this disorder ranks among cardiomyopathies also in the current definition and classification of cardiomyopathies [1, 2].

Tachycardia-induced cardiomyopathy is a disease with attributes of dilated cardiomyopathy that develop as a consequence of persistent tachycardia. It is characterized by systolic ventricular dysfunction and dilatation with heart failure symptoms that occur as a result of long-term tachycardia of either supraventricular or ventricular origin. This disease should be also considered as a cause of ventricular dysfunction in the absence of tachycardia at the time of patient presentation since the tachyarrhythmia could disappear spontaneously before the initiation of patient examination, while the hemodynamic and especially structural changes of the heart induced by long-term tachycardia may persist even weeks after arrhythmia disappearance and/or rate control achievement.

The key feature of tachycardia-induced cardiomyopathy is the reversibility of both functional and structural changes as soon as the heart rate/rhythm is well controlled. In such case, improvement or even complete functional and structural normalization may be found. A correct diagnosis is thus often stated retrospectively based on the observation of ventricular systolic function improvement and regression of ventricular dilatation after appropriate rate/rhythm control.

2. Incidence, prevalence and prognosis

Although tachycardia-induced cardiomyopathy is considered to be a relatively rare instance, its precise incidence is not described well yet. In fact, this disease is very likely to be underdiagnosed in the clinical practice despite that the link between tachycardia and dilated cardiomyopathy pattern has been known for a long time [3-5]. One reason for its underestimation may be the uncertainty whether the detected tachycardia is the primary cause of the cardiomyopathy, or whether it is rather a consequence of cardiomyopathy of different origin.

Tachycardia-induced cardiomyopathy may develop at any age. It has been documented in fetuses with persistent supraventricular tachycardias [6], in children and adolescents [7] as well as in adults [8].

Virtually, any type of arrhythmia is capable of inducing ventricular dysfunction or cardiomyopathy; however, supraventricular arrhythmias are the most commonly reported causes of tachycardia-induced cardiomyopathy. It has been predominanly described in association with atrial fibrillation, but other supraventricular arrhythmias may lead to this pathology too. Tachycardia-induced cardiomyopathy may also develop as a result of persistent ventricular tachycardia, rapid atrial and/or ventricular pacing or as a consequence of some extracardiac diseases that are associated with persistent tachycardia (Table 1). Importantly, it may also occur in patients with "only" frequent ventricular premature beats [9].

Atrial fibrillation (the most frequently reported arrhythmia associated with tachycardia-induced cardiomyopathy development) is a frequent type of supraventricular tachycardia

http://dx.doi.org/10.5772/60716

Supraventricular arrhythmias	Atrial fibrillation [13, 73]
	Atrial flutter [14, 74]
	Focal atrial tachycardia [15, 16]
	AVNRT [17, 18]
	AVRT [19, 75]
	Permanent junctional reciprocating tachycardia (PJRT) [20]
Ventricular arrhythmias	Frequent ventricular premature beats (VPBs) [9, 76]
	Idiopathic right or left ventricular outflow tract tachycardia [7, 8]
	Bundle-branch reentry ventricular tachycardia [77]
Cardiac pacing	Atrial pacing at high rates [30]
	Ventricular pacing at high rates [32]
Extracardiac causes	Thyreotoxicosis [78]
	Glucagonoma [79]
Myocarditis [80]	

Table 1. Disorders associated with tachycardia-induced cardiomyopathy development (adapted from [81])

in patients with dilated cardiomyopathy and heart failure. It appears that there is a close relationship between atrial fibrillation and heart failure: heart failure progression supports electrical and structural remodeling of the heart, which finally leads to atrial fibrillation development. On the other hand, epidemiological studies have demonstrated that patients with atrial fibrillation are at higher risk of heart failure [10] and that abnormal left-ventricular systolic function is 2.5 times more likely in elderly patients (> 65 years) with atrial fibrillation than in those without this arrhythmia [11]. In addition, sinus rhythm restoration or adequate rate control of ongoing arrhythmia are associated with the improvement or even normalization of left-ventricular ejection fraction in some of these patients. These findings indicate that at least in some cases, left-ventricular dysfunction is primarily caused by rapid heart rate during atrial fibrillation rather than by preexisting dilated cardiomyopathy. Moreover, some studies indicate that approximately 25–50% of patients with atrial fibrillation, who simultaneously suffer from ventricular dysfunction, have some degree of tachycardia-induced cardiomyopathy [12, 13].

Another instance of tachyarrhythmia that used to be associated with a relatively higher prevalence of cardiomyopathy pattern is **atrial flutter**. Some observational studies indicated that left-ventricular systolic dysfunction is present in up to 25% of patients reported to atrial flutter ablation, and in more than half of these, it is possible to observe a significant improvement or even normalization of ejection fraction during the first twelve months after successful elimination of the tachycardia [14].

Prevalence of ventricular dysfunction is relatively high also in incessant **atrial tachycardia,** since it has been reported in approximately 10–19% of cases [15, 16]. It seems that children are more susceptible to tachycardia-induced cardiomyopathy than adults. Among adults, tachycardia-induced cardiomyopathy appears to be present more often in younger adult patients with persistent atrial tachycardia than in those of a higher age, although the lower prevalence in the older population may be partially caused by difficulties to distinguish the effect of tachycardia alone from that of the underlying heart disease with regard to the systolic ventricular function. Interestingly, elimination of the arrhytmia leads to the restoration of left-ventricular function in up to 97% [16].

Supraventricular reentrant tachycardias (atrioventricular nodal reentry tachycardia (AVNRT) and atrioventricular reciprocating tachycardia (AVRT)) have usually only paroxysmal nature. If persistent, these may also induce cardiomyopathy and heart failure that are reversible after catheter ablation [17-20].

Ventricular tachycardias are usually associated with some forms of underlying structural heart diseases. Therefore, it is difficult to distinguish whether and to what extent is the observed systolic ventricular dysfunction caused by the primary disease, and how much has persistent tachycardia contributed to its severity. This may be determined more precisely in patients with idiopathic ventricular tachycardias, which (if persistent or repetitive enough) may lead to cardiomyopathy. Restoration of normal systolic performance of the left ventricle has been described in patients with successful elimination of both right-ventricular outflow tract tachycardia [8] and left-ventricular outflow tract tachycardia [7].

However, cardiomyopathy with or without symptomatic heart failure may be present also in patients with "only" **frequent premature beats.** It has been described mainly in patients with frequent ventricular ectopy [9, 21-23], but high burden of atrial premature beats may also lead to reversible cardiomyopathy [24, 25]. A prospective multicenter study that included patients with reduced left-ventricular ejection fraction due to suspected ventricular premature beat-associated cardiomyopathy has found that both systolic function and neurohumoral response (levels of natriuretic peptide) improve as soon as the ectopy is successfully eliminated and that the extent of improvement is comparable between patients with and without known structural heart disease [26]. These authors suggested that the higher the burden of ventricular premature beats (VPB), the higher the probability of systolic function improvement after ectopy elimination, with 13% baseline VPB burden being 100% sensitive and 85% specific to predict left-ventricular ejection fraction increase by ≥5% after elimination of the ectopic focus. Although not confirmed in all studies [26], some researchers have also suggested that the QRS duration of VPB is an important factor in the development of cardiomyopathy, with wider QRS complexes more likely to lead to cardiomyopathy pattern with a lower total burden of PVBs [27, 28] and that epicardial origin of VPBs is also associated with delayed LV function recovery [29].

Prognosis of dilated cardiomyopathy may vary depending on the cause. Tachycardia-induced cardiomyopathy ranks among forms of dilated cardiomyopathy with (if treated appropriately) generally good prognoses. Although studies describing recovery of patients with tachycardia-induced cardiomyopathy after sinus rhythm restoration or rate control include only small samples of patients, it appears that these causal therapeutic options may result in an improvement of left-ventricular function, positive change in neurohumoral cascade (reduced levels of natriuretic peptides) [26] and that it is likely to be linked to a generally good prognosis of tachycardia-induced cardiomyopathy.

http://dx.doi.org/10.5772/60716

3. Pathogenesis

Our current knowledge about the pathogenesis of tachycardia-induced cardiomyopathy is predominantly based on animal models that have been introduced to study heart failure [30-35]. In these experiments, heart failure is induced by rapid cardiac pacing of certain duration, at the atrial and/or ventricular level. Hemodynamic changes that result from such pacing strongly resemble findings in humans [31-35]. Similar abnormalities have been also identified in animals with "only" ventricular premature beats delivered artificially in bigeminal pattern, and these changes are reminiscent of those in humans as well [36]. Observations proving that all these alterations are fully or at least partially reversible with cessation of tachycardia also correspond with results found in humans [32, 37].

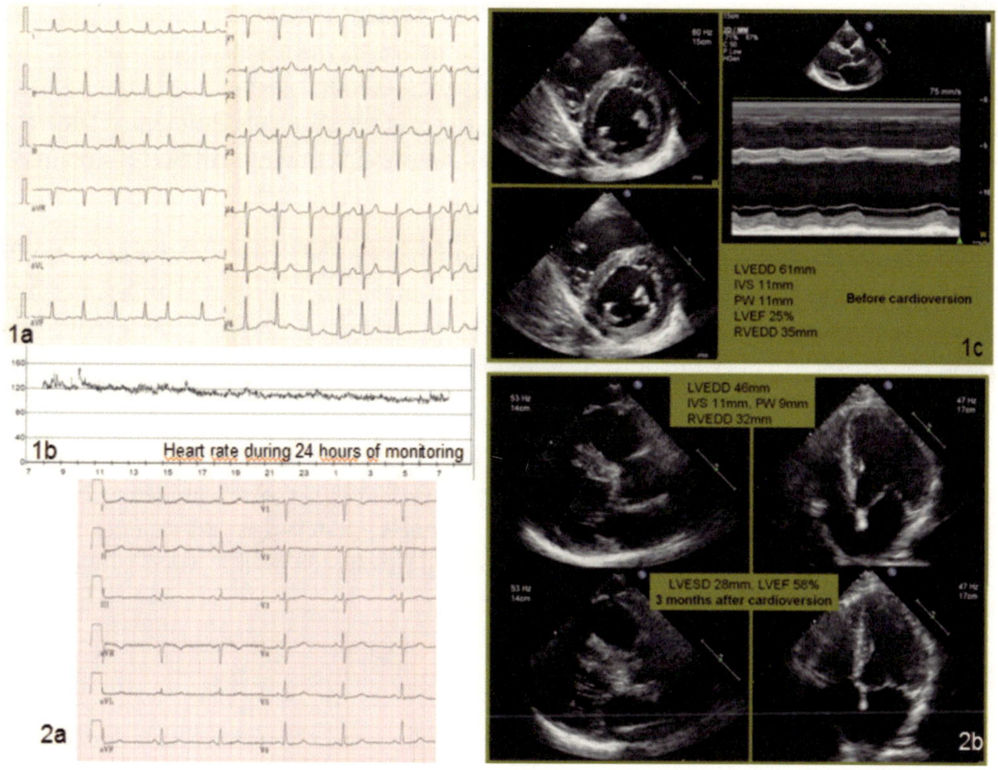

Figure 1. Tachycardia-induced cardiomyopathy in a 38-years old male with no previous history of any heart disease or arrhythmia. First episode of persistent atrial fibrillation with rapid heart rate (1a, 1b) in his life caused progressive deterioration of ventricular systolic function leading to clinical manifestation of heart failure during 4 weeks. 1c shows significantly reduced ejection fraction of the left ventricle with its incipient enlargement during the tachycardia. Both heart failure symptoms and left-ventricular systolic function rapidly improved during the following 3 weeks after sinus rhythm restoration (2a). Size and systolic function of the left ventricle then almost normalized in the horizon of 3 months after the tachycardia termination (2b).

3.1. Hemodynamic changes

Rapid atrial or ventricular pacing in experimental models leads to biventricular systolic and diastolic dysfunctions that occur relatively early after the onset of tachycardia [38, 39]. Typical findings include reduced systolic function of both ventricles reaching up to 55%, decline in cardiac output, elevation of ventricular filling pressures, systemic vascular resistance as well as ventricular systolic wall stress [33-35, 40, 41]. Systolic ventricular dysfunction is caused by the loss of contractility. In addition, contractile reserve in response to volume, inotropic agents or post-extrasystolic potentiation is affected [42, 43] and myocardial relaxation is impaired [44]. As a consequence of altered hemodynamic situation, mitral regurgitation may develop in longer-term perspective that leads to volume overload of the failing heart [45].

3.2. Structural changes

Persistent tachycardia, either induced artificially by chronic cardiac pacing or resulting from persistent tachyarrhythmia, finally leads to the dilatation of all cardiac chambers. Left ventricle increases both its end-systolic and end-diastolic volume (with end-systolic volume being affected more [33, 34]) and it further changes its geometry to a spherical shape [46]. This dilatation is usually associated with wall thinning or preservation of wall thickness without either increased heart weight or hypertrophy [45, 46].

On microscopical level, remodeling of both cardiomyocytes and extracellular matrix may be detected: disruptions of sarcolemma-basement membrane interface, myofibrillar misalignment, cellular elongation and myocyte loss (up to 39% of the total myocyte mass) have been found [40, 47, 48]. Architecture of the extracellular matrix is usually remarkably modified as well and this also contributes to myocyte misalignment and adversely affects force coupling and transmission.

In addition to functional and structural changes, electrophysiologic remodeling has been documented. Abnormal functioning of calcium channels, stretch-sensitive channel dysfunction and other abnormalities often affect and prolong repolarization that can finally result in ventricular tachycardias manifestation [49].

3.3. Neurohumoral changes

Similar to other forms of heart failure, marked neurohumoral activation occurs and leads to elevated plasma levels of natriuretic peptides, epinephrine, norepinephrine, aldosterone and renin activity [39]. Downregulation of beta-1 receptor density with the resulting decrease in beta-adrenergic responsiveness have been found as well [50, 51].

All the above-mentioned hemodynamic, structural and neurohumoral changes have been demonstrated also in humans, which supports the conclusion that pacing-induced model of heart failure could be a useful tool to study pathogenesis of tachycardia-induced cardiomyopathy.

3.4. Pathophysiology of tachycardia-induced cardiomyopathy

The development of tachycardia-induced myocardial dysfunction appears to be a result of multiple factors. Various alternations of neurohumoral and cellular activation have been identified; however, it is still uncertain whether they represent the causal factor of the functional and subsequent structural changes in all cases, or whether they are rather a consequence of tachycardia. Although the precise mechanism behind contractile dysfunction with the resulting structural changes is not fully understood yet, the research has focused mainly on three potential factors: *1) depletion of high-energy stores in the myocardium with impaired energy utilization, 2) myocardial ischemia and 3) abnormality in calcium handling.*

On subcellular level, persistent tachycardia leads to energy-stores depletion, which is associated with the reduction of adenosin-triphosphate (ATP), phosphocreatinine and creatinine levels in the myocardium. In addition, a reduced activity of the Na/K-ATPase pump has been described [52, 53a, 53b]. It is very likely due to enhanced activity of Krebs cycle oxidative enzymes and mitochondrial injury [40, 41].

Similar findings have been described in the case of myocardial ischemia. In the ischemic model, rapid depletion of energy-stores and left-ventricular dysfunction occur shortly after vessel occlusion [54]. However, their return to normal values lasts mostly about days long after the ischemic attack, which also corresponds with findings in tachycardia-induced cardiomyopathy where altered hemodynamic and structural changes resolve in prolonged time interval. Proceeding from these facts, myocardial ischemia is considered to be a potential factor that contributes to the tachycardia-induced cardiomyopathy development. In fact, abnormal coronary flow and changed ratios of subendocardial and subepicardial flow have been observed in tachycardia-induced cardiomyopathy [55, 56].

The hypothesis that abnormal handling of calcium plays a role in the genesis of tachycardia-induced cardiomyopathy has received substantial support, because the severity of calcium cycling abnormalities has been shown to correlate with the extent of ventricular dysfunction [41]. Abnormal calcium handling occurs already in the first 24 hours of rapid cardiac pacing and it may persist for more than 4 weeks after tachycardia termination [41]. Altered functions of calcium channels and transport system of the sarcoplasmatic reticulum have been identified [41, 57] and they may thus contribute to myocardial dysfunction observed in tachycardia-induced cardiomyopathy due to lower calcium availability to myocytes with the resulting contractility reduction. Some other studies suggest altered calcium-sensitivity and excitation-contraction coupling [57, 58].

An observation that tachycardia-induced cardiomyopathy does not evolve in every patient with the same type, duration and rate of a tachycardia implies *possible genetic predisposition* of some patients to develop a dilated cardiomyopathy pattern during tachycardia. In fact, one study [59] suggests that polymorphism in angiotensin-converting enzyme (ACE) gene may be involved, since one type of such polymorphism (which is associated with higher serum levels of ACE) is more frequently linked to idiopathic and ischemic cardiomyopathy manifestation. Looking at the prevalence of this polymorphism among 20 patients with tachycardia-induced cardiomyopathy as compared to another sample of 20 patients without this pattern, the authors reported a higher detection of this ACE polymorphism in the cardiomyopathic group [59].

3.5. Course of the changes over time and their reversibility

Experimental studies demonstrate that changes of hemodynamics with the reduction of cardiac output or altered systemic arterial pressure occur already in the first 24 hours of rapid pacing [32]. When continued, fast cardiac pacing then induces an elevation of ventricular filling pressures, pulmonary artery pressure and a decrease of systemic arterial pressure that reach certain plateau after one week, while cardiac output, volumes and ejection fraction deteriorate continually for 3–5 weeks with the final end-stage heart failure development [35, 45].

Cessation of tachycardia results in a resolution of these changes: in the first 48 hours after termination of cardiac pacing, a significant improvement of cardiac output, systemic vascular resistance, mean arterial pressure and filling pressures are present [39]. Left-ventricular ejection fraction also improves dramatically and normalizes within 1–2 weeks [39]. All hemodynamic variables normalize within the horizon of four weeks after tachycardia interruption, but diastolic dysfunction remains detectable even after the first month period. Importantly, elevated end-diastolic and end-systolic volumes are still present after twelve weeks of pacing discontinuation, which is consistent with substantial ventricular remodeling [33, 46], that requires longer time for its resolution.

Although the hallmark of tachycardia-induced cardiomyopathy is an improvement or even normalization of cardiac function and size with the resulting disappearance of heart failure symptoms after cessation of tachycardia or rate control achievement, there is growing evidence that the ultrastructural abnormalities of the myocardium and residual contractility dysfunction may persist. This has already been suggested in the experimental studies [53b], but similar conclusions have also been made in clinical observational reports [60, 61]. In one of these studies, ventricular function has been assessed using specle tracking and contrast-enhanced MRI with ventricular T1 mapping used as an index of diffuse fibrosis. Although the ejection fraction normalized three months after a successful ablation of initial tachycardia already, it has been possible to detect a somewhat greater indexed end-diastolic and end-systolic volume of the left ventricle in patients with tachycardia-induced cardiomyopathy as compared to healthy controls. Moreover, patients with previous tachycardia-induced cardiomyopathy have demonstrated reduced global left-ventricular corrected T1 time that implies a diffuse fibrosis [61]. In addition, another study [60] suggests that tachycardia tends to recur in some patients initially diagnosed with tachycardia-induced cardiomyopathy pattern and this recurrence of arrhythmia leads to a new decline of systolic ventricular function. Moreover, sudden death may occur in some of these patients despite normal or almost normal systolic function during the last evaluation [60].

4. Clinical manifestation and diagnosis

It is important to consider tachycardia-induced cardiomyopathy in all cases as a possible cause of systolic dysfunction and manifest heart failure, especially in patients with a new or worsened ventricular systolic dysfunction or in cases with their uncertain duration in which persistent tachycardia is found simultaneously. Since contractile dysfunction and structural

http://dx.doi.org/10.5772/60716

changes may persist even weeks after the rhythm/rate correction, tachycardia-induced cardiomyopathy should be considered as a probable reason of ventricular dysfunction and dilatation in any patient presenting with dilated cardiomyopathy pattern, despite that the initial rhythm is not pathological or the heart rate is well controlled.

Generally, persistent tachycardia (i.e. tachycardia lasting usually weeks or months) predisposes an individual to ventricular dysfunction and dilatation development, regardless of the rhythm disturbance characteristics. However, the resulting degree of systolic dysfunction and heart dilatation, the rate of their progression and the reversibility of hemodynamic and structural abnormalities after rhythm/rate correction are partially dependent on the heart rate, type and duration of the tachycardia and also on the concomitant presence of other heart diseases. In addition, there is growing evidence that irregularity of the rhythm alone may contribute to these changes manifestation and that it may also affect the rate and the extent of their resolution after rhythm correction.

Heart rate is apparently one of the most important factors. Tachycardia-induced cardiomyopathy is rate dependent: tachycardias with higher rates manifest themselves usually earlier than those with slower rates [31, 62]. In an experimental setting, pacing at slower rate or for a shorter time usually yields a lesser degree of left-ventricular systolic dysfunction [39, 63]. However, some observational studies imply that tachycardia-induced cardiomyopathy may be found more often in patients with a slower heart rate than in those with a higher rate. This was reported in retrospective observational studies that included patients referred to catheterization ablation of focal atrial tachycardia [15, 16]. Tachycardia-induced cardiomyopathy was present in 9–19% of these cases, more frequently in patients with heart rate of less than 120 bpm. Possible explanation for this finding may include the fact that faster tachycardia is associated with early symptom manifestation in form of palpitation, whereas tachycardias with lower heart rate are better tolerated by the patient, so the remodeling and signs of heart failure have enough time to develop before the patient visits a doctor.

How fast does the tachycardia have to be to induce tachycardia-induced cardiomyopathy is still not clear. Basically, any rhythm with the rate exceeding 100 bpm for a longer period of time may lead to this pathology. In this context, it is important to note that heart rate (especially in atrial fibrillation) may vary significantly as a result of physical or mental activity, i.e. patients may show well-controlled heart rate at rest that increases abnormally during minimal exercise. Therefore, Holter ECG monitoring may be useful to identify such behavior and to raise suspicion of tachycardic origin of an observed ventricular dysfunction. Cut-offs for adequate rate control have been derived from atrial fibrillation patients. They generally vary with age, but heart rate ranging between 60 and 80 bpm at rest and 90–115 bpm during a moderate exercise are usually considered as adequate (so-called strict rate control) [64]. These target rates are sometimes difficult to achieve, however. A lenient rate control strategy [65] aiming at resting heart rate <110 bpm seems to have similar long-term results as the strict rate control of atrial fibrillation and is thus preferred nowadays.

In the experimental model, persistent **ventricular tachyarrhythmias induce** generally **more significant ventricular dysfunction** than supraventricular tachycardias [38].

Tachycardia-induced cardiomyopathy may develop in a variable time-horizon since the tachycardia onset (even after many months). Together with heart rate and type of the arrhythmia, the **tachycardia duration** is responsible for the severity and reversibility of ventricular systolic dysfunction [31] as it has been discussed earlier.

Tachycardia-induced cardiomyopathy can be present as either sole pathology or it **may accompany another heart disease**. It means that the presence of other structural heart disease does not exclude concurrent presence of tachycardia-induced cardiomyopathy. In these cases, tachycardia may worsen the pre-existing ventricular dysfunction and dilatation [12]. The degree of a ventricular dysfunction is then usually inadequate to the severity of the underlying heart disease (i.e. atherosclerotic changes of the coronary arteries). Tachycardia-induced cardiomyopathy is highly probable especially in patients with recently normal systolic function of the ventricles and in those with an improvement of dysfunction after the achievement of an adequate rate/rhythm control.

Another factor which appears to contribute to tachycardia-induced cardiomyopathy is the **irregularity** of a rhythm. It is based not only on the observations that frequent ectopic supraventricular or ventricular beats are able to induce the pattern of reversible dilated cardiomyopathy [9, 22, 24], but also on studies on rate control in atrial fibrillation [66], which demonstrate that the irregularity of a fast rhythm may worsen cardiac function whereas it does not cause any significant hemodynamic worsening if the heart rate of the irregular rhythm falls generally within a normal range.

Assessment of a patient with suspected tachycardia-induced cardiomyopathy includes a detailed history and physical examination with the subsequent laboratory and imaging tests to state the diagnosis and severity of the disease.

4.1. Symptoms and signs

The manifestation of tachycardia-induced cardiomyopathy is various. The most common symptoms include palpitations and signs of heart failure. Palpitations resulting from either high rate or irregularity of the arrhythmia are often the dominant complaint of a patient with fast tachycardia. These patients thus often consult a doctor early in search of intervention and cardiomyopathy pattern then does not have enough time to develop. On the other hand, symptoms and signs of a heart failure may predominate in those patients who do not feel palpitation and are not aware of a rhythm disturbance. In such patients, decreased exercise capacity, fatigue or congestion may be the main complaint.

Due to the fact that acuteness of the symptoms forces a patient with rapid heart rate to seek medical help shortly after the arrhythmia onset, some scholars hypothesize that tachycardia-induced cardiomyopathy is present rather in patients with slower arrhythmias. Some clinical observations support such conclusions [15, 16]: The first retrospective observational study [16] included a sample of 331 patients without structural heart diseases who underwent ablation of atrial tachycardia. Tachycardia-induced cardiomyopathy was present in 9% of them and affected rather younger patients (mean age 39 vs. 51 years), more often males (60% versus 38%) with incessant or very frequent paroxysmal tachycardia (100% vs. 20%) with a slower heart rate (120 bpm vs. 149 bpm), than arrhythmias that have not been associated with ventricular dysfunction. Similar findings have been reported also in children with persistent atrial tachycardias [15]: atrial tachycardia originating within the atrial appendage was more often associated with slower heart rate (<120 bpm) at examination, asymptomatic course (75% versus 25%) and higher prevalence of tachycardia-induced cardiomyopathy as compared to atrial tachycardia of other origins.

In all other aspects, tachycardia-induced cardiomyopathy resembles other forms of dilated cardiomyopathy: symptoms and signs of heart failure, their severity as well as neurohumoral activation are principally similar.

4.2. Diagnosis

As soon as tachycardia-induced cardiomyopathy is suspected, tests that aim to confirm the diagnosis take place.

All patients should have **12-lead ECG** to document basic heart rhythm and its rate at patient presentation. Especially in cases with persistent atrial tachycardia, it is helpful to compare recent ECG tracing with an older one (if available) to distinguish whether the current P wave morphology corresponds with the documented sinus rhythm morphology or if it is rather suggestive for atrial focus. Since the heart rate may change over time, due to mental or physical activity, patients with suspected tachycardia-induced cardiomyopathy should undergo **continuous ECG monitoring** for at least 24 hours (ambulatory Holter ECG monitoring or in-patient telemetry). If uncertainty regarding the underlying rhythm persists, electrophysiologic testing should be considered.

Besides arrhythmia detection, the presence of left-ventricular dysfunction with/without ventricular dilatation should be documented. With this regard, **transthoracic echocardiography** represents a gold standard. Morphological findings are principally similar as in the dilated cardiomyopathy of other origins and differentiation between tachycardia-induced cardiomyopathy and other forms of dilated cardiomyopathy is generally not possible based on the echocardiographic pattern only, although left-ventricular end-diastolic diameter tends to be usually smaller in cases of tachycardia-induced cardiomyopathy [67].

Despite that the patient presents with tachyarrhythmia, other reasons of dilated cardiomyopathy pattern should be therefore considered as soon as the ventricular dysfunction and dilatation is documented at any imaging modality. Adult patients are thus often indicated to coronary angiography to exclude the most common substrate of ventricular dysfunction, i.e. a significant underlying coronary artery disease. History of alcohol intake, drug abuse, cancer and its treatment, thyreopathy or other metabolic or congenital disease should be searched for further.

A single-center experience suggests that also **serial NT-pro BNP** measurement may be useful to distinguish between tachycardia-induced cardiomyopathy and cardiomyopathies due to structural heart disease [68]. This study included patients who presented with supraventricular tachycardia and reduced left-ventricular ejection fraction <40% and underwent cardioversion. The NT-pro BNP level has initially been elevated in all patients. After a successful cardioversion, NT-pro BNP has decreased in virtually all patients, but the decrease has been quicker in tachycardia-induced cardiopmyopathy patients. Therefore, the ratio between the baseline NT-pro BNP and NT-pro BNP after one week following cardioversion ≥ 2.3 has had 90% sensitivity, 95% specificity and 90% accuracy to predict tachycardia-induced origin of ventricular dysfunction based on these authors.

5. Therapy

Therapeutic approach to the tachycardia-induced cardiomyopathy includes two steps: 1. tachyarrhythmia correction as it represents causal therapeutic intervention and 2. heart failure treatment.

Due to the potential reversibility of hemodynamic and structural changes in tachycardia-induced cardiomyopathy, all efforts should be made to achieve **heart rate correction or appropriate rate control.** Rhythm or rate control may be achieved using both pharmacological and non-pharmacological tools. Depending on the type of arrhythmia and presence/absence of concomitant structural heart disease, various antiarrhytmic drugs may be used to terminate the arrhythmia or to achieve adequate rate control. Especially, betablockers and class III antiarrhythmics play an irreplaceable role regarding this treatment. It is very important to avoid drugs with higher pro-arrhythmic effect (e.g. flecainide) in the presence of systolic dysfunction or drugs that may contribute to further progression of systolic dysfunction (e.g. disopyramide). Most arrhythmias that lead to tachycardia-induced cardiomyopathy are currently treatable using catheterization ablation, success rate of which reaches 60–90% depending on the type of arrhythmia. This therapeutic approach should be therefore considered as a first-line treatment in the absence of contraindication.

In atrial fibrillation, rate and rhythm control strategy have been shown to be comparable with respect to quality of life, mortality or stroke rate [64, 69]. The decision to favor rhythm control over rate control should thus be made on an individual basis, and discussed with the patient [70]. In case rate control strategy is chosen, repeated long-term ECG monitoring is instrumental to decide whether the selected treatment is appropriate and ensures acceptable rate control (strict rate control requires 60–80 bpm at rest and 90–115 bpm at moderate exercise; lenient rate control requests resting rate < 110 bpm). Atrial arrhythmias are often refractory to antiarrhythmic drugs and an acceptable rate control may be then achieved only with higher doses of AV nodal blocking agent. In such cases, catheter ablation is an option. By other supraventricular tachyarrhythmias, which lead to tachycardia-induced cardiomyopathy, restoration of sinus rhythm is usually preferred. Rhythm correction may be achieved through either pharmacological or electrical cardioversion or (preferably) via catheter ablation of the arrhythmia in these patients.

In rare cases, failing to restore sinus rhythm (even using catheter ablation) and to achieve adequate ventricular control, an ablation of AV node with insertion of a permanent pacemaker may be considered. Because of the present ventricular dysfunction prior to pacemaker insertion, biventricular systems are usually favored [71].

Treatment of heart failure symptoms due to tachycardia-induced cardiomyopathy includes standard regimen and drug spectrum as in heart failure of other origin, i.e. ACE inhibitors, beta-blockers, angiotensin-receptor blockers, diuretics and digoxin.

6. Risk of tachycardia-induced cardiomyopathy recurrence

Similarly as in the experimental models, improvement of ventricular systolic function may be often found in one week horizon and full recovery (including chamber size reduction), usually over a time period of 4–6 weeks after rhythm/rate correction. In some patients, size of the left ventricle may remain slightly enlarged [72].

Although there are no recommendations regarding follow-up of the patients who once experienced tachycardia-induced cardiomyopathy, it is advisable to observe such patients closely for at least one or two years after the initial manifestation. The reason for it is certain, although not specifically determinable risk of arrhythmia recurrence that may induce new and rapid decrease of left-ventricular ejection fraction despite cardiomyopathy could develop within months during the initial episode. Patients experiencing the recurrence of tachycardia-induced cardiomyopathy are at higher risk of sudden death [72] and implantation of an ICD may be thus considered in these cases.

7. Conclusion

The difficulties to differentiate reliably between tachycardia-induced cardiomyopathy and other forms of dilated cardiomyopathy, and the fact that the correct diagnosis is often established only retrospectively based on the improved systolic function after heart rate correction are the two most important reasons why the real prevalence of tachycardia-induced cardiomyopathy may be much higher than it is currently reported. Since it is a potentially reversible cause of heart failure, it is very important to always consider this option in the concomitant presence of dilated cardiomyopathy pattern and persistent tachycardia. An early heart rate intervention may then have substantial clinical impact.

Although experimental studies helped us to understand the basic pathophysiologic process behind the tachycardia-induced cardiomyopathy development, there is still a number of questions that need to be answered. For example, it is not clear why the tachycardia-induced cardiomyopathy does not occur in all patients with persistent tachycardia of the same type and heart rate. Furthermore, it is not clear whether or not are the patients who once developed tachycardia-induced cardiomyopathy in their life more susceptible to heart failure of another origin in the long-term perspective, similarly as are women with gestational diabetes more prone to develop the second type of diabetes in their future life. In addition, the exact pathophysiology behind tachycardia-induced cardiomyopathy is still not well understood. All these and other questions should therefore become the subjects of future research.

Acknowledgements

The work was supported by the Project for Conceptual Development of the Research Organization no. 00064203 from Ministry of Health, Czech Republic.

Author details

Lucie Riedlbauchova*

Address all correspondence to: Lucie Riedlbauchova

Section for Electrophysiology and Cardiac Pacing, Department of Cardiology, University Hospital Motol and 2nd Faculty of Medicine, Charles University in Prague, Czech Republic

References

[1] Maron BJ, Towbin JA, Thiene G, et al. Contemporary definitions and classification of the cardiomyopathies: an American Heart Association Scientific Statement from the Council on Clinical Cardiology, Heart Failure and Transplantation Committee; Quality of Care and Outcomes Research and Functional Genomics and Translational Biology Interdisciplinary Working Groups; and Council on Epidemiology and Prevention. Circulation 2006;113(14):1807–1816.

[2] Elliot P, Andersson B, Arbustini E, et al. Classification of the cardiomyopathies: a position statement from the European Society of Cardiology working group on myocardial and pericardial diseases. Eur Heart J 2008;29:270–276.

[3] Gossage AM, Braxton Hicks JA. On auricular fibrillation. QJM 1913;6:435–440.

[4] Coleman HN 3rd, Taylor RR, Pool PE, et al. Congestive heart failure following chronic tachycardia. Am Heart J 1971;81(6):790–798.

[5] Kasper EK, Agema WR, Hutchins GM, et al. The causes of dilated cardiomyopathy: a clinicopathologic review of 673 consecutive patients. J Am Coll Cardiol 1994;23(3): 586–590.

[6] Krapp M, Gembruch U, Bauman P. Venous blood flow pattern suggesting tachycardia induced cardiomyopathy in the fetus. Ultrasound Obstet Gynecol 1997;10:32–40.

[7] Singh B, Kaul U, Talwar KK, Wasir HS. Reversibility of "tachycardia induced cardiomyopathy" following the cure of idiopathic left ventricular tachycardia using radiofrequency energy. Pacing Clin Electrophysiol 1996;19(9):1391–1392.

[8] Vijgen J, Hill P, Biblo LA, Carlson MD. Tachycardia-induced cardiomyopathy secondary to right ventricular outflow tract ventricular tachycardia: improvement of left

ventricular systolic function after radiofrequency catheter ablation of the arrhythmia. J Cardiovasc Electrophysiol 1997;8(4):445–450.

[9] Baman TS, Lange DC, Ilg KJ, et al. Relationship between burden of premature ventricular complexes and left ventricular function. Heart Rhythm 2010;7(7):865–869.

[10] Stewart S, Hart CL, Hole DJ, McMurray JJ. A population-based study of the long-term risks associated with atrial fibrillation: 20-year follow-up of the Renfrew/Paisley study. Am J Med 2002;113(5):359–364.

[11] Aronow WS, Ahn C, Kronzon I. Echocardiographic findings associated with atrial fibrillation in 1699 patients aged 60 years. Am J Cardiol 1995;76:1191–1192.

[12] Redfield MM, Kay GN, Jenkins LS, et al. Tachycardia-related cardiomyopathy: a common cause of ventricular dysfunction in patients with atrial fibrillation referred for atrioventricular ablation. Mayo Clin Proc 2000;75:790–795.

[13] Edner M, Caidahl K, Bergfeldt L, et al. Prospective study of left ventricular function after radiofrequency ablation of atrioventricular junction in patients with atrial fibrillation. Br Heart J 1995;74:261–267.

[14] Pizzale S, Lemery R, Green MS, et al. Frequency and predictors of tachycardia-induced cardiomyopathy in patients with persistent atrial flutter. Can J Cardiol 2009 Aug;25(8):469–472.

[15] Sakaguchi H, Miyazaki A, Yamamoto M, et al. Clinical characteristics of focal atrial tachycardias arising from the atrial appendages during childhood. Pacing Clin Electrophysiol 2011;34(2):177–184.

[16] Medi C, Kalman JM, Haqqani H, et al. Tachycardia-mediated cardiomyopathy secondary to focal atrial tachycardia: long-term outcome after catheter ablation. J Am Coll Cardiol 2009;53(19):1791–1797.

[17] Furushima H, Chinushi M, Sugiura H, Aizawa Y. Radiofrequency catheter ablation for incessant atrioventricular nodal reentrant tachycardia normalized H-V block associated with tachycardia-induced cardiomyopathy. J Electrocardiol 2004 Oct;37(4): 315319.

[18] Selvaraj R, Ananthakrishnapillai A, Sadasivam R, Balachander J. "Pseudo PJRT"—fast-slow AV nodal reentrant tachycardia presenting with tachycardia-induced cardiomyopathy. Pacing Clin Electrophysiol 2013 Jan;36(1):e4–6. doi: 10.1111/j.1540-8159.2011.03210.x. Epub 2011 Sep 2

[19] Packer DL, Bardy GH, Worley SJ, et al. Tachycardia-induced cardiomyopathy: a reversible form of left ventricular dysfunction. Am J Cardiol 1986;57(8):563–570.

[20] Aguinaga L, Primo J, Anguera I, et al. Long-term follow-up in patients with the permanent form of junctional reciprocating tachycardia treated with radiofrequency ablation. Pacing Clin Electrophysiol 1998;21(11Pt1):2073–2078.

[21] Bogun F, Crawford T, Reich S, et al. Radiofrequency ablation of frequent, idiopathic premature ventricular complexes: comparison with a control group without intervention. Heart Rhythm 2007;4(7):863–867.

[22] Yokokawa M, Kim HM, Good E, et al. Relation of symptoms and symptom duration to premature ventricular complex-induced cardiomyopathy. Heart Rhythm 2012;9(1):92–95.

[23] Lamba J, Redfearn DP, Michael KA, et al. Radiofrequency catheter ablation for the treatment of idiopathic premature ventricular contractions originating from the right ventricular outflow tract: a systematic review and meta-analysis. Pacing Clin Electrophysiol 2014;37(1):73–78.

[24] Pacchia CF, Akoum NW, Wasmund S, Hamdan MH. Atrial bigeminy results in decreased left ventricular function: an insight into the mechanism of PVC-induced cardiomyopathy. Pacing Clin Electrophysiol 2012;35(10):1232–1235.

[25] Hasdemir C, Simsek E, Yuksel A. Premature atrial contraction-induced cardiomyopathy. Europace 2013;15:1790.

[26] Penela D, Van Huls Van Taxis C, Aguinaga L, et al. Neurohormonal, structural, and functional recovery pattern after premature ventricular complex ablation is independent of structural heart disease status in patients with depressed left ventricular ejection fraction: a prospective multicenter study. J Am Coll Cardiol 2013;62(13): 1195–1202.

[27] Carballeira Pol L, Deyell MW, Frankel DS, et al. Ventricular premature depolarization QRS duration as a new marker of risk for the development of ventricular premature depolarization-induced cardiomyopathy. Heart Rhythm 2014;11(2):299–306.

[28] Deyell MW, Park KM, Han Y, et al. Predictors of recovery of left ventricular dysfunction after ablation of frequent ventricular premature depolarizations. Heart Rhythm 2012;9(9):1465–1472.

[29] Yokokawa M, Good E, Crawford T, et al. Recovery from left ventricular dysfunction after ablation of frequent premature ventricular complexes. Heart Rhythm 2013;10(2):172–175.

[30] Whipple GH, Sheffield LT, Woodman EG, et al. Reversible congestive heart failure due to chronic rapid stimulation of the normal heart. Proc N Engl Cardiovasc Soc 1962;20:39–40.

[31] Armstrong PW, Stopps TP, Ford SE, De Bold AJ. Rapid ventricular pacing in the dog: pathophysiologic studies of heart failure. Circulation 1986;74:1075–1084.

[32] Wilson JR, Douglas P, Hickey WF, et al. Experimental congestive heart failure produced by rapid ventricular pacing in the dog: cardiac effects. Circulation 1987;75(4): 857–867.

[33] Howard RJ, Stopps TP, Moe GW, et al. Recovery from heart failure: structural and functional analysis in a canine model. Can J Physiol Pharmacol 1988;66(12):1505–1512.

[34] Morgan DE, Tomlinson CW, Qayumi AK, et al. Evaluation of ventricular contractility indexes in the dog with left ventricular dysfunction induced by rapid atrial pacing. J Am Coll Cardiol 1989;14(2):489–495.

[35] Ohno M, Cheng CP, Little WC. Mechanism of altered patterns of left ventricular filling during the development of congestive heart failure. Circulation 1994;89(5):2241–2250.

[36] Huizar JF, Kaszala K, Potfay J, et al. Left ventricular systolic dysfunction induced by ventricular ectopy: a novel model for premature ventricular contraction-induced cardiomyopathy. Circ Arrhythm Electrophysiol 2011;4(4):543–549.

[37] Damiano RJ Jr, Tripp HF Jr, Asano T, et al. Left ventricular dysfunction and dilatation resulting from chronic supraventricular tachycardia. J Thorac Cardiovasc Surg 1987;94(1):135–143.

[38] Zupan I, Rakovec P, Budihna N, Brecelj A, Kozelj M. Tachycardia induced cardiomyopathy in dogs; relation between chronic supraventricular and chronic ventricular tachycardia. Int J Cardiol 1996;56(1):75–81.

[39] Moe GW, Stopps TP, Howard RJ, Armstrong PW. Early recovery from heart failure: insights into the pathogenesis of experimental chronic pacinginduced heart failure. J Lab Clin Med 1988;112:426–432.

[40] Spinale FG, Hendrick DA, Crawford FA, et al. Chronic supraventricular tachycardia causes ventricular dysfunction and subendocardial injury in swine. Am J Physiol 1990;259:H218–H229.

[41] O'Brien PJ, Ianuzzo CD, Moe GW, et al. Rapid ventricular pacing of dogs to heart failure: biochemical and physiological studies. Can J Physiol Pharmacol 1990;68(1): 34–39.

[42] Komamura K, Shannon RP, Ihara T, et al. Exhaustion of Frank-Starling mechanism in conscious dogs with heart failure. Am J Physiol 1993;265:H1119–H1131.

[43] Spinale FG, Fulbright BM, Mukherjee R, et al. Relation between ventricular and myocyte function with tachycardia-induced cardiomyopathy. Circ Res 1992;71:174–187.

[44] Zile MR, Mukherjee R, Clayton C, Kato S, Spinale FG. Effects of chronic supraventricular pacing tachycardia on relaxation rate in isolated cardiac muscle cells. Am J Physiol 1995;268:H2104–H2113.

[45] Howard RJ, Moe GW, Armstrong PW. Sequential echocardiographic-Doppler assessment of left ventricular remodelling and mitral regurgitation during evolving experimental heart failure. Cardiovasc Res 1991;25:468–474.

[46] Tomita M, Spinale FG, Crawford FA, Zile MR. Changes in left ventricular volume, mass, and function during the development and regression of supraventricular tachycardia-induced cardiomyopathy. Disparity between recovery of systolic versus diastolic function. Circulation 1991;83:635–644.

[47] Zellner JL, Spinale FG, Eble DM, Hewett KW, Crawford FA. Alterations in myocyte shape and basement membrane attachment with tachycardia induced heart failure. Circ Res 1991;69:590–600.

[48] Kajstura J, Zhang X, Liu Y, et al. The cellular basis of pacing-induced dilated cardiomyopathy. Myocyte cell loss and myocyte cellular reactive hypertrophy. Circulation 1995;92:2306–2317.

[49] Pak PH, Nuss HB, Tunin RS, et al. Repolarization abnormalities, arrhythmia and sudden death in canine tachycardia-induced cardiomyopathy. J Am Coll Cardiol 1997;30(2):576–584.

[50] Marzo KP, Frey MJ, Wilson JR, et al. Beta-adrenergic receptor-G protein-adenylate cyclase complex in experimental canine congestive heart failure produced by rapid ventricular pacing. Circ Res 1991;69(6):1546–1556.

[51] Yonemochi H, Yasunaga S, Teshima Y, et al. Rapid electrical stimulation of contraction reduces the density of beta-adrenergic receptors and responsiveness of cultured neonatal rat cardiomyocytes. Possible involvement of microtubule disassembly secondary to mechanical stress. Circulation 2000;101(22):2625–2630.

[52] Moe GW, Montgomery C, Howard RJ, et al. Left ventricular myocardial blood flow, metabolism, and effects of treatment with enalapril: further insights into the mechanisms of canine experimental pacing-induced heart failure. J Lab Clin Med 1993;121(2):294–301.

[53] (a) Spinale FG, Clayton C, Tanaka R, et al. Myocardial Na+, K(+)-ATPase in tachycardia induced cardiomyopathy. J Mol Cell Cardiol 1992;24(3):277–294. (b) Spinale FG, Holzgrefe HH, Mukherjee R, et al. LV and myocyte structure and function after early recovery from tachycardia-induced cardiomyopathy. Am J Physiol 1995;268:H836–H847.

[54] Reimer KA, Hill ML, Jennings RB. Prolonged depletion of ATP and of the adenine nucleotide pool due to delayed resynthesis of adenine nucleotides following reversible myocardial ischemic injury in dogs. J Mol Cell Cardiol 1981;13(2):229–239.

[55] Spinale FG, Tanaka R, Crawford FA, Zile MR. Changes in myocardial blood flow during development of and recovery from tachycardia-induced cardiomyopathy. Circulation 1992;85:717–729.

[56] Shannon RP, Komamura K, Shen YT, et al. Impaired regional subendocardial coronary flow reserve in conscious dogs with pacing-induced heart failure. Am J Physiol 1993;265:H801–H809.

[57] Perreault CL, Shannon RP, Komamura K, et al. Abnormalities in intracellular calcium regulation and contractile function in myocardium from dogs with pacing-induced heart failure. J Clin Invest 1992;89(3):932–938.

[58] Wolff MR, Whitesell LF, Moss RL. Calcium sensitivity of isometric tension is increased in canine experimental heart failure. Circ Res 1995;76:781–789.

[59] Deshmukh PM, Krishnamani R, Romanyshyn M, et al. Association of angiotensin converting enzyme gene polymorphism with tachycardia cardiomyopathy. Int J Mol Med 2004;13(3):455–458.

[60] Nerheim P, Birger-Botkin S, Piracha L, Olshansky B. Heart failure and sudden death in patients with tachycardia-induced cardiomyopathy and recurrent tachycardia. Circulation 2004;110(3):247–252.

[61] Ling LH, Kalman JM, Ellims AH, et al. Diffuse ventricular fibrosis is a late outcome of tachycardia-mediated cardiomyopathy after successful ablation. Circ Arrhythm Electrophysiol 2013;6(4):697–704.

[62] Ravens U, Davia K, Davies CH, et al. Tachycardia-induced failure alters contractile properties of canine ventricular myocytes. Cardiovasc Res 1996;32(3):613–621.

[63] Redfield MM, Aarhus LL, Wright RS, Burnett JC, Jr. Cardiorenal and neurohumoral function in a canine model of early left ventricular dysfunction. Circulation 1993;87:2016–2022.

[64] AFFIRM Investigators. A comparison of rate control and rhythm control in patients with atrial fibrillation. N Engl J Med 2002;347:1825–1833.

[65] Van Gelder IC, Groenveld HF, Crijns HJ, et al. Lenient versus strict rate control in patients with atrial fibrillation.N Engl J Med 2010;362:1363–1373.

[66] Melenovsky V, Hay I, Fetics BJ, et al. Functional impact of rate irregularity in patients with heart failure and atrial fibrillation receiving cardiac resynchronization therapy. Eur Heart J 2005 Apr;26(7):705–711.

[67] Jeong YH, Choi KJ, Song JM, et al. Diagnostic approach and treatment strategy in tachycardia-induced cardiomyopathy. Clin Cardiol 2008;31(4):172–178.

[68] Nia AM, Gassanov N, Dahlem KM, et al. Diagnostic accuracy of NT-proBNP ratio (BNP-R) for early diagnosis of tachycardia-mediated cardiomyopathy: a pilot study. Clin Res Cardiol 2011;100(10):887–896.

[69] Roy D, Talajic M, Nattel S, et al. Rhythm control versus rate control for atrial fibrillation and heart failure. N Engl J Med 2008;358:2667–2677.

[70] Camm AJ, Kirchhof P, Lip GY, et al. Guidelines for the management of atrial fibrillation: the Task Force for the Management of Atrial Fibrillation of the European Society of Cardiology (ESC). Eur Heart J 2010 Oct;31(19):2369–2429.

[71] Brignole M, Auricchio A, Baron-Esquivias G, et al. 2013 ESC guidelines on cardiac pacing and cardiac resynchronization therapy: the task force on cardiac pacing and resynchronization therapy of the European Society of Cardiology (ESC). Developed in collaboration with the European Heart Rhythm Association (EHRA). Europace 2013 Aug;15(8):1070–1118.

[72] Dandamudi G, Rampurwala AY, Mahenthiran J, et al. Persistent left ventricular dilatation in tachycardia-induced cardiomyopathy patients after appropriate treatment and normalization of ejection fraction. Heart Rhythm 2008;5(8):1111–1114.

[73] Brill IC. Auricular fibrillation with congestive failure and no other evidence of organic heart disease. Am Heart J 1937;13:175–182.

[74] David M, Rothman S, Shapiro T. First reported case of recurrent tachycardia-induced cardiomyopathy due to atrial flutter. QJM 2014 May;107(5):383–386.

[75] Cheruvu C, Walker B, Kuchar D, Subbiah RN. Successful ablation of incessant AV reentrant tachycardia in a patient on extracorporeal membrane oxygenation. Heart Lung Circ 2014 Jan;23(1):e12–5. doi: 10.1016/j.hlc.2013.06.011. Epub 2013 Aug 6.

[76] Chugh SS, Shen WK, Luria DM, Smith HC. First evidence of premature ventricular complex-induced cardiomyopathy: a potentially reversible cause of heart failure. J Cardiovasc Electrophysiol 2000;11(3):328–329.

[77] Singh B, Sudan D, Kaul U. Radiofrequency ablation for bundle branch reentrant tachycardia in a patient with aortic valve replacement and left ventricular dysfunction. Indian Heart J 1998;50(5):551–553.

[78] Yu YH, Bilezikian JP. Tachycardia-induced cardiomyopathy secondary to thyrotoxicosis: a young man with previously unrecognized Graves' disease. Thyroid 2000;10(10):923–927.

[79] Chang-Chretien K, Chew JT, Judge DP. Reversible dilated cardiomyopathy associated with glucagonoma. Heart 2004;90(7):e44.

[80] Cognet T, Lairez O, Marchal P, et al. A family history of dilated cardiomyopathy induced by viral myocarditis. Case Rep Cardiol 2012;2012:204371. doi: 10.1155/2012/204371. Epub 2012 Feb 27.

[81] Khasnis A, Jongnarangsin K, Abela G, et al. Tachycardia-induced cardiomyopathy: a review of literature. Pacing Clin Electrophysiol 2005 Jul;28(7):710–721.

Chapter 5

The Trigeminocardiac Reflex — An Example of Reflexive Heart Rhythm Change

Tumul Chowdhury, Belachew Arasho, Nora Sandu,
Cyrill Meuwly and Bernhard Schaller

Additional information is available at the end of the chapter

http://dx.doi.org/10.5772/60215

Abstract

The trigeminocardiac reflex (TCR) is defined as the sudden onset of parasympathetic dysrhythmia, sympathetic hypotension, apnoea or gastric hyper-motility during mechanical/thermal stimulation of any of the sensory branches of the trigeminal nerve. The risk factors that are already known for increasing the prevalence of the TCR include anatomical location, hypercapnia, hypoxemia, light general anaesthesia, age (more pronounced in children), the nature of the provoking stimulus (stimulus strength and duration) and different drugs. Already different potential confounders are also identified. This discussion about risk factors has its importance because of the substantial consequences for functional outcome after intraoperative TCR occurrence. But there remains still a substantial lack of thorough understanding of the TCR, the current treatment options for patients with TCR include a mostly empirical approach: (i) risk factor identification and modification; (ii) prophylactic measures of vital signs and (iii) administration of vagolytic agents or sympathomimetics. In this context, we have now created different thinking models so that we can preoperatively plan a skull base surgery procedure safely in relation to a potential occurrence of the TCR episodes. This chapter provides an overview of this unique reflex that presents a unique interaction between heart and brain. In addition, this also illustrates the mechanism of various cardiac rhythm changes related to the TCR.

Keywords: Atropine, trigeminocardiac reflex, oculocardiac reflex, skull base surgery, treatment, trigeminal nerve, study design, evidence

INTECH
open science | open minds

1. Introduction

The fifth cranial nerve is the largest of all the cranial nerves and provides sensory supply to the face, scalp, sinus and mucosa of the nose and mouth as well as the dura mater of the middle, anterior and part of the posterior cranial fossa [1–3]. Stimulation of any of these sensory parts of trigeminal nerve has been shown to initiate the trigeminocardiac reflex (TCR) and also produce various cardiac arrhythmias besides other less life-threatening symptoms [1, 3, 4, 5]. Initially, this reflex has been studied in animals and is therefore known for more than a century [6–8], under the term of "trigemino-respiratory reflex" and now its revival as sudden infant death syndrome (SIDS). In the early 20th century, the TCR has gained much clinical and less experimental attention in the form of the oculocardiac reflex (OCR) which is the predominant cardiac response associated with the stimulation of the ophthalmic division of the trigeminal nerve during ocular surgeries [9, 10]. Then later, Schaller et al., for the first time, demonstrated that the TCR occurred with the stimulation of the intracranial portion of the trigeminal nerve as well [1]. In addition, Schaller and his group later sub-summarized all these reflexes under the term TCR [2, 11], what is now generally accepted. Since then, there have been extensive discussions about the reflex itself, about the prophylaxis or risk factors, about treatment and about the influence of the TCR on functional outcome when it occurs during the intracranial or the extra-cranial procedures. Schaller and his group could demonstrate the ubiquitary occurrence of this reflex in any skull base procedure during 20 last years.

The TCR also serves as an important interaction between brain and heart, and thus provides deeper understanding of mechanisms related to various cardiac changes related to various extra/intracranial surgeries [4, 12–16]. The TCR represents as a model for different other diseases like, for example, sudden infant death syndrome (SIDS). Therefore, this chapter highlights the various aspects of TCR including its definition, epidemiology, risk factors and management. Special consideration is given to illustrate the mechanism of various cardiac rhythm changes related to the TCR.

2. Definition and pathophysiology of the trigeminocardiac reflex

Since its first description in 1999, the TCR is defined as the sudden onset of parasympathetic dysrhythmia, sympathetic hypotension, apnoea or gastric hyper-motility during stimulation of any of the sensory branches of the trigeminal nerve [1]. The proposed underlying mechanism for the development of the TCR is that the sensory nerve endings of the trigeminal nerve send neuronal signals via the Gasserian ganglion to the sensory nucleus of the trigeminal nerve, forming the afferent pathway of the reflex arc [1, 2]. This afferent pathway continues along the short internuncial nerve fibres in the reticular formation of the pons to connect with the efferent pathway in the motor nucleus of the vagus nerve in the nucleus ambiguus (see Figure 1) [1]. Since this initial description, nearly all trigeminal innervated structures except Meckel's cave have been reported to lead to a TCR. Several lines of experimental evidence demonstrate that trigeminal induced cardiovascular reflexes could be excitatory evoked initially in the trigemi-

http://dx.doi.org/10.5772/60215

nal nucleus caudalis and subsequently in the parabrachial nucleus, the rostral ventrolateral medulla oblongata, the dorsal medullary reticular field and the paratrigeminal nucleus [3, 17, 18]. Even so several studies on cellular level were performed, the exact cellular mechanism remains still to be explored.

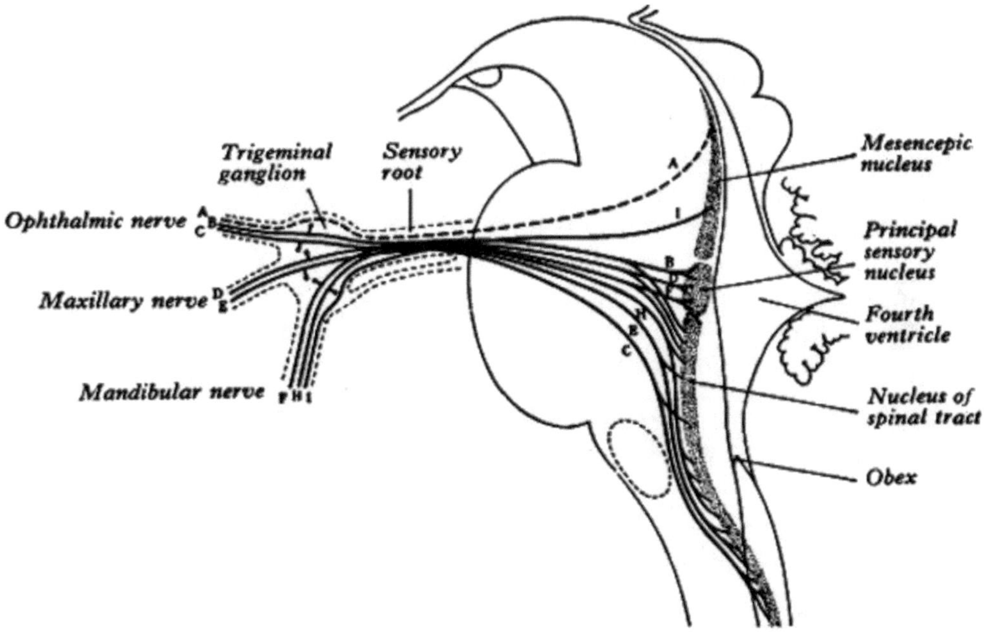

Figure 1. Trigeminal nerve with trigeminal ganglion and nuclei (from Warwick, R, Williams PL. Gray`s Anatomy, 35th ed., p 1001, Edinburgh, Churchill Livingstone, 1973)

According to the current knowledge, the TCR occurs during the peripheral and central manipulations of the trigeminal nerve as well as around Ganglion Gasseri manipulation. The OCR, which is an accepted peripheral sub-form of the TCR, has been reported in patients with ocular surgeries and consecutive trigeminal nerve manipulations since several decades [9, 10, 19]. After 1999, as Schaller et al., for the first time, reported the occurrence of the TCR in skull base and neurological surgeries, it was thought that OCR and TCR are both the same reflex [1]. The underlying cellular mechanism is not yet fully understood (see Figure 2), but is believed to be the same as the TCR reported earlier on in more detail during activation of the central or intracranial portions of the trigeminal nerve [2].

3. Epidemiology of the trigeminocardiac reflex

The TCR occurs with mechanical/thermal manipulation around any of the branches of the trigeminal nerve [9, 10, 19–23], with specific prevalence in specific anatomical locations [1]. The OCR being a sub-variant of the peripheral TCR is studied extensively earlier and was said to occur in up to 67% after ophthalmic surgery [24]. Because of publication bias, the real prevalence may be substantially smaller, even the peripheral TCR has generally a higher prevalence than the central TCR. According to the senior author Schaller's experience, the central TCR occurs in up to 10–18% of the patients [1, 25–27]. In a retrospective time-series review of 125 patients operated for tumours of the cerebello-pontine angle, Schaller et al. noticed the TCR occurrence in 11%. [4] Three of these patients in this series developed asystole which lasted from 30 to 70 seconds [1]. In contrast to earlier studies on OCR, Schaller – for the first time – took into consideration both the heart rate and blood pressure and defined TCR as heart rate and mean arterial blood pressure (MABP) 20% lower than the baseline [1].

In another retrospective time-series study, Schaller also showed the TCR occurrence during microvascular decompression of the trigeminal nerve for trigeminal neuralgia [27]. In this review on 28 patients, the prevalence of TCR was up to 18% with the same definition used as in his prior above-mentioned study [27]. TCR was also reported during transsphenoidal surgery for pituitary adenoma [11, 26, 28]. Among 117 patients who underwent transsphenoidal surgery for pituitary adenoma, 10% developed a TCR during the surgical procedure [26]. Peripheral stimulation of the nasopharynx may also lead to (peripheral) TCR [11].

In several other neurosurgical procedures, there exists only case reports or small case series, so that a robust prevalence of TCR occurrence is not (yet) known.

4. Heart and the trigeminocardiac reflex

The TCR is a clinical phenomenon that reflects interactions of many organs to the brain [4, 12, 14, 19, 29–31]. Among all the organs, the connection between heart and brain is unique and presents a wide array of clinical manifestations when the TCR gets incited [16]. These clinical signs include drop in heart rate and blood pressure, asytole, ventricular tachycardia/fibrillation, ST-T wave changes and other forms of arrhythmias [4, 5, 12–16, 29, 31–65]. Stimulus especially in form of stretch has found to be the strongest inciting factor for the TCR [1]. However, mild stimulus may also results into TCR episodes [3, 18, 35]. Chowdhury et al. reported that mild stimulus in the form of skin closure could able to produce transient asystole and questioned about the severity of stimulus and TCR manifestation. In another report, Chowdhury et al. further suggested that various manifestations of TCR episodes (bradycardia, hypertension, asystole) as well as different subtypes of TCR (peripheral and central) could manifest in the same patient [4, 13]. Again, in this report, transient asystole manifested during the skin closure as well [4]. Author postulated that the different sympathetic outflow responses could be due to different depths of anaesthesia, which coupled with different forms of TCR stimulation probably contributed to different haemodynamic responses in the same patient and obscured the classical manifestation of TCR [3]. Strikingly, the cardiovascular changes of TCR phenomenon mainly reported due to acute stimulation (peri-operatively) of trigeminal nerve; however, Chowdhury and Schaller highlighted the first description of chronic form of TCR [40].

As highlighted in a review by Chowdhury et al., the other rare cardiac perturbation i.e. coronary spasm in neurosurgical patients may be the mere manifestation of TCR events [16].

http://dx.doi.org/10.5772/60215

In this case series review, author found that in most of the neurosurgical conditions, dural stimulation provoked the ST-T wave changes, ventricular tachycardia and ventricular fibrillation [16]. The vagal mediated acetylcholine receptors have been also linked with the development of spasm [16]. Though majority of coronary spasm events were of transient nature (few minutes to few hours); however, very few of them also developed perioperative myocardial infarction.

5. Risk factors for occurrence of the trigeminocardiac reflex

Because of the still fragmented knowledge about the TCR and the consecutive limited therapeutic options, the risk factors gain increased importance. However, it is best known that such risk factors are not easy to proof in retrospective studies as they are predominantly available in TCR research. The risk factors already known to increase the incidence of TCR include (i) hypercapnia, (ii) hypoxemia, (iii) light general anaesthesia, (iv) age (more pronounced in children), (v) the nature of the provoking stimulus (stimulus strength and duration) and (vi) drugs. Recent systematic reviews, however, have identified several potential co-founders for these mentioned risk factors. Drugs known to increase the TCR include (i) potent narcotic agents (sufentanil and alfentanil) [66, 67], (ii) beta-blockers and (iii) calcium channel blockers [68]. Narcotics may augment vagal tone through their inhibitory action on the sympathetic nervous system [1, 69–71]. Beta-blockers reduce the sympathetic response of the heart and, by so doing, augment the vagal cardiac response resulting in bradycardia. Calcium channel blockers result in peripheral arterial smooth muscle relaxation and vasodilatation causing reduction in blood pressure. In patients undergoing trigeminal manipulations, this worsens the vagal effect that occurs in some patients. In previous publications about the TCR, the study design (mostly case control) may have led to different bias regarding the risk factors [39], such as recall bias and non-response bias to only mention two examples. From this point of view, a randomized controlled trial or a systematic review are requested to show best a cause-and-effect relationship for the risk factors.

In the recent years, it has more and more raised the question if the main search on risk factors is not a too linear thinking to overcome the complexity of the TCR. However, we think that risk factors are still an important key to better understand the TCR; even these risk factors have led to the development of the thinking model of TCR rather than to direct treatment consequences.

6. Clinical significance of the trigeminocardiac reflex and why it should be treated

Most authors recognized that the TCR is a transient, but potentially life-threatening response to any manipulation of the fifth cranial nerve subsiding with latency after cessation of the stimulus. But, in case of the development of severe bradycardia and asystole, the administration of peripheral muscarinic acetylcholine receptor blockage at the heart is warranted in addition to cessation of the stimulus. Even so often mentioned, but still not understood from all: The vagal blockage potential of atropine is only insufficient for the prevention of hypotension or bradycardia.

Rath et al. reported a case of asystole occurring in a patient who was undergoing percutaneous retrogasserian glycerol rhizolysis for trigeminal neuralgia [72]. Immediately after the injection of anhydrous glycerol, the patient became unresponsive; the pulse became impalpable, blood pressure unrecordable, the ECG showed asystole and had a respiratory arrest. The patient regained consciousness and heart rate and blood pressure returned to normal after 30 seconds with oxygen and IV atropine [72]. Prabhakar et al. also reported a case of sudden asystole without prior bradycardia which occurred during surgery for cerebellopontine angle tumour [72]. This case was just managed by cessation of the manipulation without the administration of vagolytic agents [74]. Fayol et al. also reported a five-year-old boy who was operated for strabismus and possibly died due to OCR which developed on underlying myocarditis [74]. These cases demonstrate the (clinical) importance of the TCR which may range from mild bradycardia which responds to simple cessation of the stimulus to asystole and severe bradycardia requiring additional intervention with vagolytics. In some rare but serious cases, it may lead to death if not detected early and appropriate measures taken.

In addition, hypotension which occurs during the TCR may lead to myocardial and cerebral hypoperfusion/infarction in those who are at risk for these conditions. It has also been shown that the hypotension may lead to worse functional outcomes in hearing/vestibular function in patients operated for vestibular schwannoma compared to those who do not develop the reflex [25, 75]. In a prospective study of 100 patients after vestibular schwannoma surgery, Gharabaghi et al. found out that the occurrence of TCR was 11% [25]. With an overall hearing preservation of 47%, 11.1% of the patients in the TCR group and 51.4% of those in the non-TCR group experienced preserved hearing function postoperatively [25]. In addition, in cases involving larger tumours, an intraoperative TCR was associated with a significantly worse postoperative hearing function during vestibular schwannoma surgery suggesting that the hypotension following TCR is – in addition to the tumor size – a negative prognostic factor for hearing preservation in patients undergoing VS surgery [25]. In another study, Schaller et al. compared the occurrence and persistence of tinnitus in patients with and without TCR [76]. Among 36 patients operated for vestibular schwannoma, TCR occurred in 17% and influenced the occurrence of postoperative ipsilateral tinnitus: The overall incidence of postoperative ipsilateral tinnitus was 22%. A total of 60% patients in the TCR subgroup and only 17% of in the non-TCR subgroup experienced ipsilateral tinnitus postoperatively [76]. These studies show that there is a tendency for increased complication rates in patients who developed TCR compared to those without it, again stressing the importance of looking it carefully during neurosurgical and especially skull base surgical procedures.

7. Management of the trigeminocardiac reflex

The best and more effective treatment for TCR is still a matter of intensive debate [77–86]. It is beyond the scope of this manuscript to discuss all this in detail. Without any doubt, the application of atropine is not the only modality of treatment, based on cellular knowledge of the reflex and also based on the meanwhile extensive clinical experience. To the authors opinion, the first and the most important "management option" for the TCR is to be aware of its potential danger and to minimize any mechanical/thermal stimulation of the nerve during any interventional procedure in or around the skull base.

According to the empirical experience on the TCR, and according to the current level of evidence [87], we have summarized the current recommendation as follows [35]:

Risk factor identification and modification (*Evidence Grade D*)

Prophylactic treatment with either vagolytic agents or peripheral nerve blocks in case of peripheral manipulations of the trigeminal nerve (*Evidence Grade B–C*)

Careful cardiovascular monitoring during anaesthesia especially in those with risk factors for TCR (*Evidence Grade B–C*)

Treatment of the condition when it occurs (*Evidence Grade B–C*)

- cessation of the manipulation
- local anaesthetic infiltration or blockage of the nerve
- administration of vagolytic agents or adrenaline (peripher >> central >> Ganglion)

We can see that there is a lack of good evidence in the TCR, mostly based on the literature that is predominantly based on case reports and only seldom case-control studies. Additionally, this modest evidence is underlined by a substantial publication bias. As a consequence of this, the recommendations are more general as one might wish.

The risk of TCR, however, should be considered in any interventional procedure, especially at the skull base that takes place in trigeminally innervated structures. We have developed recently a thinking model that would give a preoperative idea about the risk of the TCR that can be expected in surgery in a specific neuroanatomical region [36]. If any mechanical stimulation to the trigeminal nerve is necessary, which is a rather "robust" nerve, it should be as gentle as possible. We have now different preoperative thinking models [36, 37] that should help the surgeon as well the anaesthetics to delimit the intraoperative occurrence of the TCR before operation and to perform adapted precautions. These manoeuvres should help to further decrease the incidence of the TCR.

If working in the vicinity of the trigeminal nerve or its branches, there should be an intensive communication between surgeon and anaesthesist. From our experience, this is perhaps one of the key factors of success. Continuous intraoperative haemodynamic monitoring has been shown to be an appropriate medium to interrupt any interventional manoeuvres immediately upon the first signs of occurrence of TCR. This technique has been proven to be sufficient to return to normal haemodynamic levels without the necessity of additional (anticholinergic) medication, if the cessation of stimulus was within a considerable time span before postoperative persistent neurological deficits occur [77, 78]. Following this empiric strategy, an uneventful further intraoperative and postoperative course may be achieved.

If controlled arterial hypotension is already preoperatively planned to be performed during the interventional procedure, the prophylaxis of TCR is better accomplished with local anesthetic infiltration or block of the nerve(s) which convey afferent stimuli leading to the reflex. Shende et al. studied the efficacy of peribulbar block with bupivacaine in patients operated for retinal detachment [79]. They collected 60 patients who were randomly assigned to receive either bupivacaine or IV morphine and studied the incidence and severity of the OCR. Apart from significantly reducing the incidence of OCR (30% vs 70%), peribulbar bupivacaine also attenuated the severity of the reflex [79]. Gupta et al. studied the effect of peribulbar block in comparison to topical application of local anesthetic in children scheduled for strabismus surgery. They found out that the incidence and severity of OCR intraoperatively was significantly reduced in children who received a peribulbar block [80]. Misurya et al. studied the effectiveness of prophylactic intravenous atropine sulphate which blocks the peripheral muscarinic receptors at the heart and retrobulbar xylocaine hydrochloride, which blocks the conduction at ciliary ganglion on the afferent limb of OCR. In this study, both atropine and retrobulbar xylocaine reduced the rate of OCR to 10–20%. But, when both methods were used together, they were able to completely suppress the OCR [81].

If there is no contraindication to intravenous anticholinergics, atropine and/or glycopyrrolate IV may be used to partially prevent a TCR [82]. Hunsley et al. evaluated the efficacy of IV atropine and glycopyrrolate in the prevention of the OCR in children operated for strabismus. They tested different doses of the two drugs, glycopyrrolate 5 and 7.5 mg/kg and atropine 10 and 15 mg/kg. Overall, there is a reduction in the rate of bradycardia by 23.8–33.3% [83]. But these authors noticed that even higher doses of the two drugs, atropine 15mg/kg and glycopyrrolate 7.5mg/kg i.v., given 5 min before induction of anesthesia, are not sufficient to protect completely against the OCR in children. In a study done to evaluate the efficacy of IV or IM vagolytic agents (atropine and glycopyrrpolate) in children undergoing squint surgery, Mirakhur et al. evaluated them in a controlled study and found out that the administration of the anticholinergic agents in both the IV and the IM forms may decrease the occurrence of the OCR [84]. The overall frequency was approximately 40% (62 of 160 patients), but was 90% in those patients who did not receive anticholinergic drugs [84]. The authors concluded that the administration of anticholinergic drugs, even by the IM route, decreased the frequency, and glycopyrrolate 10 mg per kg being the most efficacious by this route [84]. As consequences of this literature and our own experience, the administration of anticholinergics has shown to be ineffective in completely preventing the TCR [73, 88]. The use of atropine is, nowadays, therefore questioned because cholinergic blockage reduces but does not totally prevent either bradycardia or hypotension in animals [85]. Another reason is that a trigeminal depressor response includes both the activation of vagal cardioinhibitory fibres and the inhibition of adrenergic vasoconstriction as demonstrated after electrical stimulation of the spinal trigeminal tract and trigeminal nuclear complex. In addition, atropine may cause serious cardiac arrhythmias itself, especially when halothane is the primary anaesthetic agent and hence the dose must be carefully chosen [86]. Prabhakar et al., for example, reported a 48-year-old female who developed severe bradycardia and hypotension during craniotomy for parietal convexity meningioma; she was unresponsive to atropine and successfully managed with epinephrine [89]. The action of adrenaline is to increase peripheral resistance via alpha-1 adrenoceptor vasoconstriction, so that blood is shunted to the body core, and the alpha-1 adrenoceptor response which is to increase cardiac rate and output [89]. This important case report underscores the fact that TCR may be refractory to atropine and other vagolyticse and may rather need to be managed with epinephrine [89]. One the other hand, the personal experience with atropine is, besides its potential danger as described already earlier, that if given prophylactic in cases of risk for the occurrence of TCR it leads to a smaller change in TCR haemodynamic. In this context, the recently developed different thinking models help to better plan already preoperatively the procedure. This discussion about smaller haemodynamic changes has gained more and more importance during the last years, because of the functional outcome that is influenced by the TCR.

From our experience, the treatment of TCR deserves more attention in the daily practice. If a TCR is elicited, the underlying stimulus has to be stopped until the haemodynamic disturbances have been recovered to normal values. Any occurrence of the TCR corresponds to the intensity of the mechanical/thermal stimulation on the sensory part of the fifth nerve. From own and other clinical experience, abrupt and sustained traction is more likely to evoke the TCR than smooth and gentle manipulations [32–34, 78].

8. Recommendation from our practice

What makes us different from others? "Not a lot" is the answer. We use the same medication and the same procedures as in other large centres and as recommended here. These differences are only small and irrelevant to us. But we have highly standardized operative and anesthesiological processes [90–92]. This takes, for example, into consideration the relevant risk factors of TCR for skull base surgery. By this high standardization, we can reach also a high resilience of our processes, reflecting in the relative low prevalence of TCR compared to other centres [91, 93-95]. We have already previously summarized our recommendations [35] (Figure 2)

9. View to the future

The research on the TCR is now on a crossroad [39]. We have had a relative long phase in which case report and small case series have given substantial input to the development of the research on this topic. This research method has led to several biases in the TCR research: first in the prevalence and second in the risk factor, to mention only those both with that are mostly affected. This will be still needed in the future, of course, but we should now think to other research methods that lead to better evidence. In the first phase of TCR research, there were a lot of opinions that have led now to several really good systematic reviews that have created facts or at least trends. But starting from this newly created knowledge, there were now published several thinking models of the TCR to overcome on the one hand the complexity of information that is now available on this topic by generalizing and to make accurate forecast of risk for a specific operation. Such models helps us to better organize the information that is available and therefore make better decisions for our patients and adopt more effective treatment strategies. This new phase of TCR research has once again revolutionized the

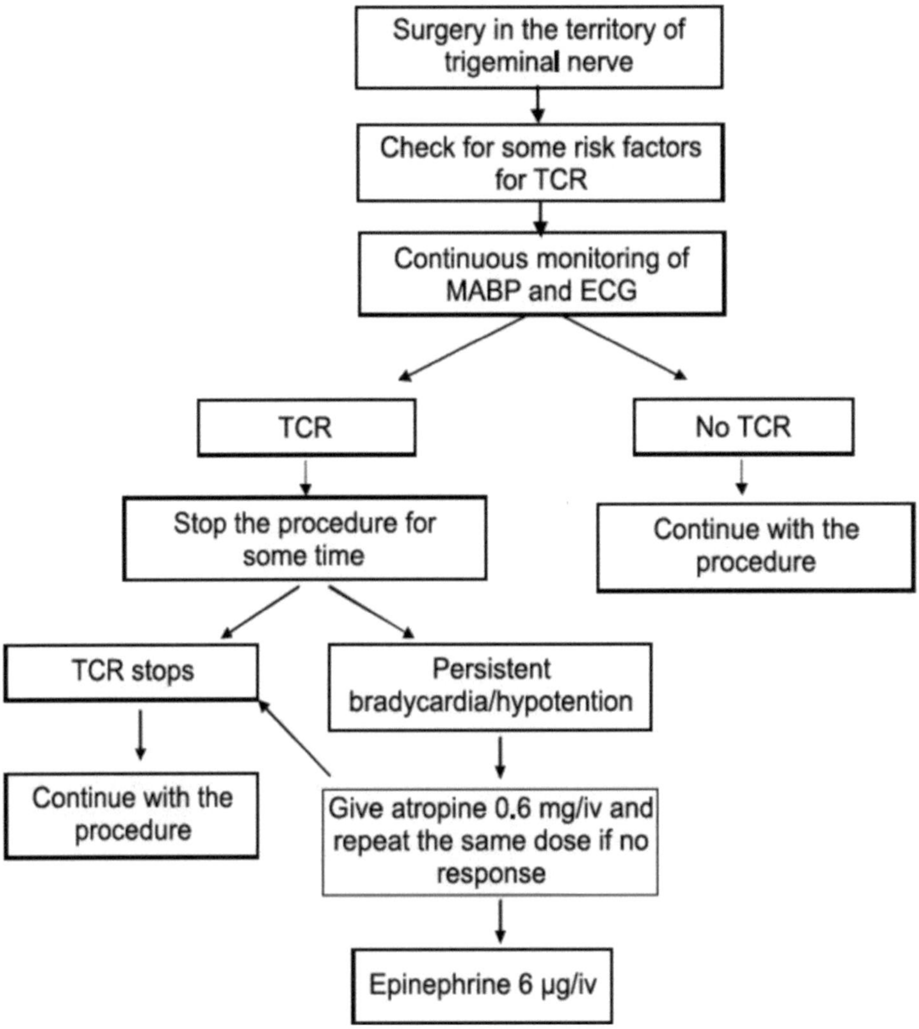

Figure 2. Treatment recommendation for trigeminocardiac reflex[35].

importance of the TCR: It is now possible to preoperatively have a really good risk stratification of the occurrence of the TCR.

These thinking model have certainly to be checked out and adapted when needed in the future [see for example 37], but we have now a good basis canalize and generalize our information and knowledge. This will lead that the TCR goes away from an interesting and important phenomenon to a real and important fact of the skull base surgery.

Following the increasing complexity of our today's hospitals, there is also the need to adapt the TCR prevalences to the new reality. It is and remains, without any doubt, important to uncover risk factors and to make root analysis of TCR occurrence. But in a next step, we have also to look on what is going well in the non-TCR cases and to uncover what makes

http://dx.doi.org/10.5772/60215

the processes robust and resilient. This will be going up from a TCR-research I to a TCR-research II.

10. Conclusion

In the present paper, we illustrated the clinical relevance of the TCR on skull base surgery as well as neuroscience and discussed its management. Further clinical studies may help to describe the only partly understood reflex arc in more details on the one hand and to develop more precise prophylactic as well as intraoperative treatment options on the other hand. Such more expensive study designs will lead to better evidence in different aspects of the TCR research. But we have currently already good tools, like several thinking models that help, for example, to have already preoperatively an idea about the potential prevalence of TCR occurrence in a specific region of surgery and in specific patients. To additionally better understand the resilience of the non-TCR cases will further help to better understand the complexity of TCR occurrence and open the door for TCR research II. Anyway it will be exciting to follow the further research on this interesting and important topic of skull base surgery

Author details

Tumul Chowdhury[1], Belachew Arasho[2], Nora Sandu[3], Cyrill Meuwly[4] and Bernhard Schaller[3,5*]

*Address all correspondence to: bernhardjschaller@gmail.com

1 University of Manitoba, Canada

2 University of Addis Abbeba, Ethiopia

3 University of Southampton, UK

4 University of Basel, Switzerland

5 University of Lille, France

References

[1] Schaller B, Probst R, Strebel S, Gratzl O. Trigeminocardiac reflex during surgery in the cerebellopontine angle. J Neurosurg 1999;90:215-20.

[2] Schaller B. Trigeminocardiac reflex: A clinical phenomenon or a new physiological entity? J Neurol 2004;251:658-65.

[3] Schaller B, Cornelius JF, Prabhakar H, Koerbel A, Gnanalingham K, Sandu N, et al. The trigeminocardiac reflex: An update of the current knowledge. J Neurosurg Anesthesiol 2009;21:187-95.

[4] Chowdhury T, Sandu N, Meuwly C, Cappellani RB, Schaller B. Trigeminocardiac reflex: Differental behaviour and risk factors in the course of the trigeminal nerve. Future Neurolgy 2014;9:41-7.

[5] Chowdhury T, Sandu N, Schaller B, Meuwly C. Peripheral trigeminocardiac reflex. Am J Otolaryngol 2013;34(5):616.

[6] Kratschmer F. Ueber Reflexe von der Nasenschleimhaut auf Athmung und Kreislauf. Sber Akad Wiss Wien 1870;62:147-70.

[7] Kratschmer F. On reflexes from the nasal mucous membrane on respiration and circulation. Translated by E. Ullmann. Respir Physiol 2001;127:93-104.

[8] Widdicombe J. Reflexes from the lungs and airways: Historical perspectives. J Appl Physiol 2006;101:628-34.

[9] Ashner B. Über einen bisher noch nicht beschriebenen Reflex, vom Auge auf Kreislauf und Atmung. Verschwinden des Radialispulses bei Druck auf das Auge. Wien Klin Wochenschr 1908;21:1529-30.

[10] Dagnini G. Interno ad un reflesso provocato inalcuni emplegica collo stimolo della come e colla pressione sul bulbo oculare. Bull Sci Med (Bologna) 1908;8:380.

[11] Schaller BJ, Filis A, Buchfelder M. Trigemino-cardiac reflex in humans initiated by peripheral stimulation during neurosurgical skull-base operations. Its first description. Acta Neurochir (Wien) 2008;150:715-8.

[12] Chowdhury T, Sandu N, Sadr-Eshkevari P, Meuwly C, Schaller B. Trigeminocardiac reflex: current trends. Expert Rev Cardiovasc Ther 2014;12(1):9-11.

[13] Chowdhury T, Sandu N, Schaller B. New insights to the role of (Nor-)adrenaline and trigeminal cardiac reflex. In: Bennun A (ed), Adrenaline, Nova Science Publisher, New York, USA, 2014; pp 71-80.

[14] Spiriev T, Sandu N, Kondoff S, Tzekov C, Schaller B. Tic and autonomic symptoms. J Neurosurg 2012;116(6):1397-8.

[15] Spiriev T, Kondoff S, Schaller B. Cardiovascular changes after subarachnoid hemorrhage initiated by the trigeminocardiac reflex-first description of a case series. J Neurosurg Anesthesiol 2011;23(4):379-80.

[16] Chowdhury T, Meuwly C, Sandu N, Cappellani RB, Schaller B. Coronary spams in neurosurgical patients and role of trigeminocardiac reflex. Neuro Res Int 2014;2014: 974930.

[17] Ohshita N, Nakajo N, Takemura M. Characteristics of the trigeminal depressor response in cats. J Neurosci Res 2004;76:891-901.

[18] Schaller BJ, Buchfelder M. Trigemino-cardiac reflex in skull base surgery: From a better understanding to a better outcome? Acta Neurochir (Wien) 2006;148:1029-31.

[19] Alexander JP. Reflex disturbances of cardiac rhythm during ophthalmic surgery. Br J Ophthalmol 1975;59:518-24.

[20] Loewinger J, Cohen M, Levi E. Bradycardia during elevation of a zygomatic arch fracture. J Oral Maxillofac Surg 1987;45:710-1.

[21] Barnard NA, Bainton R. Bradycardia and the trigeminal nerve. J Craniomaxillofac Surg 1990;18:359-60.

[22] Roberts RS, Best JA, Shapiro RD. Trigeminocardiac reflex during temporomandibular joint arthroscopy: Report of a case. J Oral Maxillofac Surg 1999;57:854-6.

[23] Shearer ES, Wenstone R. Bradycardia during elevation of zygomatic fractures. A variation of the oculocardiac reflex. Anaesthesia 1987;42:1207-8.

[24] Apt L, Isenberg S, Gaffney WL. The oculocardiac reflex in strabismus surgery. Am J Ophthalmol 1973;76:533-6.

[25] Gharabaghi A, Koerbel A, Samii A, Kaminsky J, Von Goesseln H, Tatagiba M, et al. The impact of hypotension due to the trigeminocardiac reflex on auditory function in vestibular schwannoma surgery. J Neurosurg 2006;104:369-75.

[26] Schaller B. Trigemino-cardiac reflex during transsphenoidal surgery for pituitary adenomas. Clin Neurol Neurosurg 2005;107:468-74.

[27] Schaller B. Trigeminocardiac reflex during microvascular trigeminal decompression in cases of trigeminal neuralgia. J Neurosurg Anesthesiol 2005;17:45-8.

[28] Filis A, Schaller B, Buchfelder M. Trigeminocardiac reflex in pituitary surgery. A prospective pilot study. Nervenarzt 2008;79:669-75.

[29] Sandu N, Abdulazim A, Spiriev T, Arasho B, Schaller B. The role of the immunoinflammatory response after cardiac arrest. Arch Med Sci. 2011;7(4):570-1.

[30] Spiriev T, Sandu N, Arasho B, Kondoff S, Tzekov C, Schaller B. A new predisposing factor for trigemino-cardiac reflex during subdural empyema drainage: a case report. J Med Case Rep. 2010;4:391.

[31] Cornelius JF, Sadr-Eshkevari P, Arasho BD, Sandu N, Spiriev T, Lemaitre F, Schaller B. The trigemino-cardiac reflex in adults: Own experience. Expert Rev Cardiovasc Ther. 2010;8(7):895-8.

[32] Schaller B, Filis A, Buchfelder M. Cardiac autonomic control in neurosurgery. Arch Med Sci 2007;4:287-92.

[33] Schaller B, Buchfelder M. Trigemino-cardiac reflex: A recently discovered "oxygen-conserving" response? The potential therapeutic role of a physiological reflex. Arch Med Sci 2006;2:3-5.

[34] Schaller B, Cornelius JF, Sandu N, Ottaviani G, Perez-Pinzon MA. Oxygen-conserving reflexes of the brain: The current molecular knowledge. J Cell Mol Med 2009;13:644-7.

[35] Arasho B, Sandu N, Spiriev T, Prabhakar H, Schaller B. Management of the trigeminocardiac reflex: facts and own experience. Neurology India 2009;57(4):375-80.

[36] Meuwly C, Golanov E, Sandu N, Schaller B. Trigeminocardiac reflex trigger point within the skull base: Anatomical perspective 2015; in press.

[37] Meuwly C, Golanov E, Chowdhury T, Erne P, Schaller B. Trigeminocardiac reflex: New thinking model about the definition based on a literature review. Medicine (Baltimore) 2015;94:e484.

[38] Meuwly C, Chowdhury T, Schaller B. Topical lidocaine to suppress trigemino-cardiac reflex. Br J Anaesth. 2013;111(2):302.

[39] Sandu N, Sadr-Eshkevari P, Schaller BJ. Usefulness of case reports to improve medical knowledge regarding trigemino-cardiac reflex in skull base surgery. J Med Case Rep. 2011;5:149.

[40] Chowdhury T, Cappellani RB, Schaller B. Chronic trigemino-cardiac reflex in patient with orbital floor fracture: Role of surgery and first description. J Neurosurg Anesthesiol 2014;26(1):91-2.

[41] Chowdhury T, Cappellani RB, Schaller B. Retrogasserian glycerol rhizolysis: First description of occurrence trigeminocardiac reflex. J Neurosurg Anesthesiol 2014;26(1): 86-7.

[42] Spiriev T, Tzekov C, Laleva L, Kostadinova C, Kondoff S, Sandu N, Schaller B. Central trigeminocardiac reflex in pediatric neurosurgery: A case report and review of the literature. J Med Case Rep. 2012;6:372.

[43] Spiriev T, Prabhakar H, Sandu N, Tzekov C, Kondoff S, Laleva L, Schaller B. Use of hydrogen peroxide in neurosurgery: Case series of cardiovascular complications. JRSM Short Rep. 2012;3(1):6.

[44] Spiriev T, Kondoff S, Schaller B. Trigeminocardiac reflex during temporary clipping in aneurismal surgery: First description. J Neurosurg Anesthesiol 2011;23(3):271-2.

[45] Spiriev T, Tzekov C, Kondoff S, Laleva L, Sandu N, Arasho B, Schaller B. Trigemino-cardiac reflex during chronic subdural haematoma removal: Report of chemical initiation of dural sensitization. JRSM Short Rep. 2011;2(4):27.

[46] Sandu N, Spiriev T, Lemaitre F, Filis A, Schaller B. New molecular knowledge towards the trigemino-cardiac reflex as a cerebral oxygen-conserving reflex. ScientificWorld Journal 2010;10:811-7.

[47] Sandu N, Cornelius J, Filis A, Nöthen C, Rasper J, Kulinsky VI, Schaller BJ. Cerebral hemodynamic changes during the trigeminocardiac reflex: Description of a new animal model protocol. ScientificWorld Journal 2010;10:1416-23.

[48] Schaller B, Probst R, Gratzl O, Rem JA, Hauser R, Tolnay M. Different aspects of hearing preservation in surgery of vestibular schwannoma in women and men. Acta Neurochir (Wien) 1996;138:1275-81.

[49] Nöthen C, Sandu N, Prabhakar H, Filis A, Arasho BD, Buchfelder M, Schaller BJ. Trigemino-cardiac reflex and antecedent transient ischemic attacks. Expert Rev Cardiovasc Ther. 2010;8(4):509-12.

[50] Schaller B, Sandu N, Cornelius JF, Filis A. Asystole due to trigemino-cardiac reflex: A rare complication of trans-sphenoidal surgery for pituitary adenoma. J Clin Neurosci. 2009;16(12):1709.

[51] Schaller B, Cornelius JF, Prabhakar H, Koerbel A, Gnanalingham K, Sandu N, Ottaviani G, Filis A, Buchfelder M. The trigemino-cardiac reflex: An update of the current knowledge. J Neurosurg Anesthesiol 2009;21(3):187-95.

[52] Schaller B, Filis A, Sandu N, Buchfelder M. Peripheral trigemino-cardiac reflex. Acta Neurochir (Wien) 2009;151(12):1727.

[53] Schaller BJ, Sandu N, Cornelius JF, Filis A, Perez-Pinzon MA. Oxygen-conserving implications of the trigemino-cardiac reflex in the brain: The molecular basis of neuroprotection? Mol Med. 2009;15(5-6):125-6.

[54] Schaller B, Sandu N, Filis A, Ottaviani G, Rasper J, Nöethen C, Buchfelder M. Trigemino-cardiac reflex: The trigeminal depressor responses during skull base surgery. Clin Neurol Neurosurg. 2009;111(2):220.

[55] Schaller B, Sandu N, Filis A, Buchfelder M. Peribulbar block or topical application of local anaesthesia combined for paediatric strabismus surgery. Anaesthesia 2008;63(10):1142-3.

[56] Schaller B, Sandu N, Filis A, Buchfelder M. Cardiovascular responses during percutaneous radiofrequency thermocoagulation therapy in primary trigeminal neuralgia: An explanation of the trigeminocardiac reflex? J Neurosurg Anesthesiol 2008;20(4): 270.

[57] Schaller B, Filis A, Sandu N, Rasper J, Noethen C, Buchfelder M. Trigemino-cardiac reflex may be refractory to conventional management in adults. Acta Neurochir (Wien) 2008 ;150(9):929-30.

[58] Schaller B, Sandu N, Ottoviani G, Filis A, Noethen C, Buchfelder M. Transient asystole during endoscopic transsphenoidal surgery: An example of trigeminocardiac reflex. Pituitary 2009;12(3):271-2.

[59] Schaller BJ, Filis A, Buchfelder M. Trigemino-cardiac reflex in humans initiated by peripheral stimulation during neurosurgical skull-base operations. Its first description. Acta Neurochir (Wien) 2008;150(7):715-7.

[60] Schaller B, Filis A, Buchfelder M. Trigeminocardiac reflex in embolization of intracranial dural arteriovenous fistula. AJNR Am J Neuroradiol 2008;29(7):E55.

[61] Schaller BJ, Rasper J, Filis A, Buchfelder M. Difference in functional outcome of ipsilateral tinnitus after intraoperative occurrence of the trigemino-cardiac reflex in surgery for vestibular schwannomas. Acta Neurochir (Wien) 2008;150(2):157-60.

[62] Filis A, Schaller B, Buchfelder M. Trigeminocardiac reflex in pituitary surgery. A prospective pilot study. Nervenarzt 2008;79(6):669-75.

[63] Schaller BJ, Weigel D, Filis A, Buchfelder M. Trigemino-cardiac reflex during transsphenoidal surgery for pituitary adenomas: methodological description of a prospective skull base study protocol. Brain Res. 2007;1149:69-7.

[64] Schaller BJ, Filis A, Buchfelder M. Detection and prevention of the trigeminocardiac reflex during skull base surgery. Acta Neurochir (Wien) 2007;149(3):33.

[65] Schaller BJ. Reflexive autonomic activation in skull base surgery. Nova Science Publisher, New York, USA, 2008; pp

[66] Rivard JC, Lebowitz PW. Bradycardia after alfentanil-succinylcholine. Anaesth Analg. 1988;76:907.

[67] Starr NJ, Sethna DH, Estafanos FG. Bradycardia and asystole following rapid administration of sufentanil with vecuronium. Anesthesiology 1986;64:521-3.

[68] Schmeling WT, Kampine JP, Warltier DC. Negative chronotropic actions of sufentanil and vecuronium in chronically instrumented dogs pretreated with propanolol and/or diltiazem. Anaesth Analg 1989;66:4-14.

[69] Blanc VF, Hardy JF, Milot J, Jacob JL. The oculocardiac reflex: A graphic and statistical analysis in infants and children. Can Anaesthet Soc J 1983;30:360-9.

[70] Lang S, Lanigan DT, Van der Wal M. Trigeminocardiac reflexes: Maxillary and mandibular variants of the oculocardiac reflex. Can J Anaesth 1991;38:757-60

[71] Moonie GT, Ress EL, Elton D. The oculocardiac reflex during strabismus surgery. Can Anaesthet Soc J 1964;11:621.

[72] Rath GP, Dash HH, Prabhakar H, Pandia MP. Cardiorespiratory arrest during trigeminal rhizolysis. Anaesthesia 2007;62:971-2.

[73] Prabhakar H, Anand N, Chouhan RS, Bithal PK. Brief report of special case: Sudden asystole during surgery in the cerebellopontine angle. Acta Neurochir (Wien) 2006;148:699-700.

[74] Fayon M, Gauthier M, Blanc VF, Ahronheim GA, Michaud J. Intraoperative cardiac arrest due to the oculocardiac reflex and subsequent death in a child with occult Epstein-Barr Virus myocarditis. Anesthesiology 1995;83:622-4.

[75] Schaller BJ. Trigeminocardiac reflex. J Neurosurg 2007;107:243.

[76] Schaller BJ, Rasper J, Filis A, Buchfelder M. Difference in functional outcome of ipsilateral tinnitus after intraoperative occurrence of the trigeminocardiac reflex in surgery for vestibular schwannomas. Acta Neurochir (Wien) 2008;150:157-60.

[77] Gharabaghi A, Acioly de Sousa MA, Tatagiba M. Detection and prevention of the trigeminocardiac reflex during cerebellopontine angle surgery. Acta Neurochir (Wien) 2006;148:1223.

[78] Koerbel A, Gharabaghi A, Samii A, Gerganov V, Von Gösseln H, Tatagiba M, et al. Trigeminocardiac reflex during skull base surgery: Mechanism and management. Acta Neurochir (Wien) 2005;147:727-33.

[79] Shende D, Sadhasivam S, Madan R. Effects of peribulbar bupivacaine as an adjunct to general anesthesia on peri-operative outcome following retinal detachment surgery. Anaesthesia 2000;55:970-5.

[80] Gupta N, Kumar R, Kumar S, Sehgal R, Sharma KR. A prospective randomised double blind study to evaluate the effect of peribulbar block or topical application of local anesthesia combined with general anesthesia on intra-operative and postoperative complications during paediatric strabismus surgery. Anaesthesia 2007;62:1110-3.

[81] Misurya VK, Singh SP, Kulshrestha VK. Prevention of oculocardiac reflex during extraocular muscle surgery. Indian J Ophthalmol 1990;38:85-7.

[82] Blanc VF. Trigeminocardiac reflexes. Can J Anesthesia 1991;38:696-9.

[83] Hunsley E, Bush GH, Jones CJ. A study of Glycopyrrolate and Atropine in the suppression of the oculocardiac reflex in strabismus surgery in children. Br J Anaesth. 1982;54:459-64.

[84] Mirakhur RK, Jones CJ, Dundee JW, Archer DB. I.M or I.V atropine or glycopyrrolate for the prevention of oculocardiac reflex in children undergoing squint surgery. Br J Anaesth 1982;54:1059.

[85] Schaller B, Sandu N, Filis A, Buchfelder M. Peribulbar block of topical application of local anesthesia combined for paediatric strabismus surgery. Anaesthesia 2008;63:1142-3.

[86] Schaller BJ, Weigel D, Filis A, Buchfelder M. Trigemino-cardiac reflex during transsphenoidal surgery for pituitary adenomas: Methodological description of a prospective skull base study protocol. Brain Res 2007;1149:1169-75.

[87] Howick Chalmers JI, Glasziou P, Greenhalgh, Heneghan TC, Liberati A, Moschetti I, Phillips B, Thornton H. "The 2011 Oxford CEBM Levels of Evidence" (Introductory Document). Oxford Centre for Evidence-Based Medicine. http://www.cebm.net/index.aspx?o=5653 (retrieved at 02.12.2014).

[88] Prabhakar H, Rath GP, Arora R. Sudden cardiac standstill during skin flap elevation in a patient undergoing craniotomy. J Neurosurg Anesthesiol 2007;19:203-4.

[89] Prabhakar H, Ali Z, Rath GP. Trigemino-cardiac reflex may be refractory to conventional management in adults. Acta Neurochir (Wien) 2008;150:509-10.

[90] Chowdhury T, Sandu N, Meuwly C, Cappellani RB, Schaller B. Trigeminocardiac reflex: Different behaviour and risk factors in the course of the trigeminal nerve. Future Neurol 2015; 9:41-7.

[91] Schaller B, Rüegg SJ. Brain tumor and seizures. Pathophysiology and its implications for treatment revised. Epilepsia 2003;44:1223-32.

[92] Schaller B, Buchfelder M. Delayed trigeminocardiac reflex induced by an intraorbital foreign body. Ophthalmologica 2006;220:348.

[93] Cornelius JF, Sadr-Eshkevari P, Arasho BD, Sandu N, Spiriev T, Lemaitre F, Schaller B. The trigemino-cardiac reflex in adults: Own experience. Exp Rev Cardiovasc Ther. 2010; 8:509-12.

[94] Sandu N, Sadr-Eshkevari P, Schaller BJ. Usefulness of case reports to improve medical knowledge regarding tirgemino-cardiac reflex in skull base surgery. J Med Case Rep. 2011;5:1-3.

[95] Sandu N, Chowdhury T, Sadr-Eshkevari P, Filis A, Arasho B, Spiriev T, Schaller B. Trigeminocardiac reflex during cerebellopontine angle surgery: Anatomical location as a new risk factor. Future Neurol 2015;10:7-13.

Section 2

Cardiac Antiarrhythmics

Chapter 6

A Review on Amiodarone as an Antiarrhythmic Drug

Fereshteh Mehraein

Additional information is available at the end of the chapter

http://dx.doi.org/10.5772/60418

Abstract

Antiarrhythmic drugs are used to suppress abnormal heart rhythms by different mechanisms. Amiodarone as an iodinated benzofuran derivative is a potent antiarrhythmic drug that is being used for the treatment of a wide variety of cardiac arrhythmias. Amiodarone has been reported to cause frequent and potentially serious toxicity. It was estimated that the prevalence of side effects was 15 % in the first year and increased to 50% with long-term therapy. Thyroid, lung, liver, ophthalmologic and neurologic systems can be affected by Amiodarone. Most of the adverse effects of the drug are related to its dosage and duration of administration. Therefore the effectiveness of Amiodarone in long-term treatment of patients with heart arrhythmia is limited because of the development of its adverse side effects.

Keywords: Antiarrhythmic drugs, Amiodarone, Side effects

1. Introduction

Antiarrhythmic drugs are used to suppress abnormal heart rhythms and have been differentiated by their antiarrhythmic action according to the classification system developed by Vaughen-Williams in 1970 [1]. The classification includes five major groups of antiarrhythmic drugs, classes I, II, III, IV and V (Table 1). Class I agents are sodium channel blockers, class II are beta blockers, class III are potassium channel blockers, class IV are calcium channel blockers and class V agents work by unknown mechanisms. The class I agents are classified into class Ia, Ib and Ic. Ia class includes Quinidine, Procainamide and Dispopyramide. They slow the rate of rise of phase 0, lengthen the refractory period and the width of the monophasic action potential. Quinidine is one of the oldest antiarrhythmic agents derived from the cinchona tree bark and has anti malarial, antipyretic and antiarrhythmic effects. Procainamide and its main metabolite, N-acetyl Procainamide are effective for treating supraventricular and ventricular arrhythmias. Disopyramide has three important side effects. It is vagolytic causing urinary retention, constipation and dry mouth. The class 1b agents are pure sodium channel blockers. This class includes Lidocaine, Phenytoin Mexiletine and Tocainide. Class Ib antiarrhythmic agents used only for the management of ventricular tachyarrhythmia. The class Ic agents are strong sodium channel blockers. This class comprises of Flecainide, Encainide, Propafenone and Moricizine. They are being used to treat ventricular and supraventricular tachyarrhythmia. They are contraindicated in patients with structural heart disease due to the risk of precipitating life-threatening ventricular arrhythmias. Class II drugs include Metoprolol, Carvedilol, Atenolol, Propranolol and Bisoprolol. They antagonize beta-receptors inhibiting the effect of the sympathetic nervous system resulting in decreased heart rate, contractility and conductivity. The class III agents are drugs that block the potassium channel as their main anti arrhythmic effect. This class includes Sotalol, Dofetilide, Ibutilide, and Amiodarone. They exert their effect by prolonging the refractory period. Sotalol is a nonspecific beta adrenergic receptor blocker with potassium channel blocking properties that is used in managing ventricular arrhythmias and atrial fibrillation. Dofetilide is a potassium channel blocker and excreted by the kidneys. Ibutilide is a short-acting intravenous potassium channel blocker that is used only for the acute termination of atrial fibrillation or flutter. Class IV drugs are Verapamil and Diltiazem. These drugs are known as nondihydropyridine and act by blocking cardiac calcium uptake. They are used to slow AV nodal conduction by decreasing heart rate. Class V agents include Adenosine, Digoxin, magnesium and sulphate are used in supraventricular arrhythmias, especially heart failure with atrial fibrillation, contraindicated in patients with ventricular arrhythmias [1–3]. Amiodarone is considered one of the most effective antiarrhythmic drugs which is widely prescribed. Here, its clinical uses as well as its side effects are reviewed.

Mechanism	Examples	Class
These drugs block cardiac sodium channels and depress phase 0 of the action potential. Class Ia drugs treat atrial fibrillation and ventricular arrhythmia.	Quinidine, Procainamide, Disopyramide	Ia
These drugs are cardiac sodium channel blockers and shorten the action potential. They are used for ventricular tachycardia.	Lidocaine, Phenytoin, Mexiletine and Tocainide	Ib
These drugs are cardiac sodium channel blockers. The class Ic drugs are commonly used to treat ventricular and supraventricular tachyarrhythmia.	Flecainide, Encainide, Propafenone and Moricizine	Ic
These drugs are known as beta-blockers and decrease heart rate, contractility and conductivity.	Metoprolol, Carvedilol, Atenolol, Ppropranolol, Bisoprolol	II
These drugs act by blocking cardiac potassium channels. They are effective to treat atrial fibrillation and ventricular tachycardia.	Amiodarone, Sotalol, Dofetilide, Ibutilide,	III
These are cardiac calcium channel blockers. They are used to slow AV nodal conduction decreasing heart rate.	Verapamil, Diltiazem	IV
unknown mechanisms	Adenosine, Digoxin, magnesium and sulfate	V

Table 1. Classification of antiarrhythmic drugs (based on mechanism of action)

2. History and main uses

Cardiac dysrhythmia also known as arrhythmia or irregular heartbeats is a group of conditions in which the electrical activity of the heart is irregular [4]. Arrhythmias may occur in the atria or ventricles [5] and is one of the most common signs of anomaly in heart function. Amiodarone as an iodinated benzofuran derivative (Figure 1) is a potent antiarrhythmic drug that is being used for the treatment of a wide variety of cardiac arrhythmias [6]. For the first time, the Russian physiologist, Gleb Von Anrep discovered the original precursor molecule of Amiodarone that was called Khellin. Khellin is the extract of an African plant named Khella. Anrep noticed that one of his technicians' angina symptom was cured after he took Khellin [7, 8]. In 1960, European pharmaceutical industries were working on the preparations of extracts derived from Khellin and finally they purified and developed Amiodarone in1961 [7]. Oral Amiodarone that suppresses life-threatening ventricular arrhythmias and also chronic atrial fibrillation is available in tablets of 200 mg and 400 mg in generic forms as Cardarone and Pacerone, respectively. In addition to the tablet forms, it is also available in solution for intravenous administration. Intravenous administration of Amiodarone is effective in suppressing serious arrhythmias which reduces the need for atrial fibrillation cardiac surgeries. The intravenous administration of Amiodarone requires following a restrict dosing schedule. Amiodarone is typically given in high doses of 800-1600 mg daily, either intravenously or orally until the arrhythmia is under control, although for long-term oral administration of the drug 200 - 600 mg daily is recommended [8–10].

3. Mechanism of action

Amiodarone is a Class III antiarrhythmic agent [7, 8] that prolongs the duration of action potential and hence increases the refractory period of atrial, nodal and ventricular tissues, thereby has a very broad spectrum of activity. An increase in the refractory period of the atrial cells is a major contributing factor for controlling the atrial tachyarrhythmia [5–7]. A reduction in the permeability of the A-V node, both anterograde and retrograde, explains the efficacy of the medicine in nodal tachycardia caused by reentry through the A-V node [11–13]. Its action on ventricular arrhythmias is explained by a number of mechanisms, e.g. its effect on the atrium and A-V node results in a reduction in the frequency of stimuli reaching the ventricle, thus giving the ventricular cell mass enough time to repolarize in cases where there have been nonsynchronous refractory periods. Furthermore, prolonging the refractory period of the His-Purkinje system and ventricular contractile fibers reduces or prevents micro reentry [5–7]. Amiodarone increases coronary blood flow, decreases cardiac oxygen requirements without producing negative inotropic effects and also suppresses ectopic pacemakers, and this is particularly valuable in arrhythmias associated with ischemic damage or angina pectoris [10 –17].

3.1. Metabolism

Amiodarone is incompletely and erratically absorbed following oral administration. Absolute bioavailability ranges from 22 to 86% but there is extensive inter-subject variations [6, 7]. Its metabolism occurs in the gut wall and in the liver that could determine the availability of the medicine. The half-life of Amiodarone is long and with chronic oral dosing can be from 14 to 110 days but is usually in the range of 14–59 days. The principal metabolite of Amiodarone, which has been detected in the plasma and other tissues, is Desethylamiodarone [16, 18]. This metabolite has been reported to have a longer half-life than Amiodarone, i.e. 10 hours after a single dose of Amiodarone and 60– 90 days after chronic dosing with Amiodarone. The mechanism of action of this metabolite is not yet known. Amiodarone is highly protein bound and is thought to bind strongly to proteins at concentrations of 10μg/mL. It is believed that most of the medicine is excreted via the liver and gastrointestinal tract by biliary excretion [16, 8]. There may be some hepatic recirculation too. The apparent volume of distribution after oral administration (200–400mg) of Amiodarone is 6.31 ± 4.93L/kg. Amiodarone is highly lipid soluble and tends to accumulate in adipose tissues as well as in highly perfused organs, e.g. lung, bone marrow, adrenals, liver, pancreas, heart, spleen and kidney. The concentration of Amiodarone in packed red blood cells is approximately 60% of that in plasma [8, 9]. Amiodarone and its metabolite Desethylamiodarone (DEA) can cross the placenta and therefore it may be toxic to embryo [8, 9]. Amiodarone is metabolized in the liver by cytochrome P450 enzyme system [8] and excreted through biliary route with almost no elimination via renal route [11, 12].

3.2. Chemistry

Amiodarone is a benzofuran derivative with two atoms of iodine per molecule (Figure 1), with a molecular weight of 645.32 g/mol, It is highly lipophilic and is not water soluble [9, 12, 13].

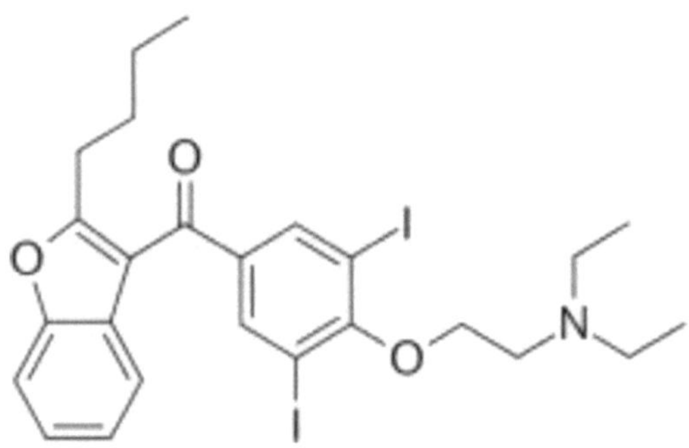

Figure 1. Chemical structure of Amiodarone

3.3. Interactions

Amiodarone is subject to multiple interactions with oral anticoagulants (e.g. Warfarin) and any drugs that cause bradycardia, e.g. beta blockers and calcium channel blockers. Amiodarone increases Digoxin level [8, 9]. Drugs that deplete potassium from the body (e.g. diuretics) should be avoided in the time of treatment with this drug. Amiodarone may increase Phenytoin levels [8, 11].

4. Side effects

Amiodarone has been reported to cause frequent and potentially serious toxicity [13, 15, 16, 18]. Most of the adverse effects of the drug are related to its dosage and duration of administration, e.g. concurrent use of other antiarrhythmic agents, severity of underlying disease state, and individual variation in pharmacokinetic profile of the medicine in each individual [11, 18]. In most patients who have been administered Amiodarone for a long period of time experienced one of the side effects [16, 18]. Even low doses of the drug are associated with significant adverse effects [18]. It was estimated that the prevalence of side effects was 15 % in the first year and increased to 50% with long-term therapy [19–21]. Thyroid, lung, gastrointestinal organs, ophthalmologic and neurologic systems can be affected by Amiodarone [16, 18].

4.1. Thyroid dysfunction

As Amiodarone may induce thyroid disorders, particularly in patients with personal history of thyroid disorders, clinical and biological monitoring recommended before starting the treatment, during the treatment and for several months after the treatment ends [21–23]. Serum TSH levels should be measured when thyroid dysfunction is suspected. Amiodarone contains two atoms of iodine per molecule (Figure 1). This amounts to 37.5% of organic iodine by molecular weight, of which 10% is deiodinated to yield free iodine. It has the potential to cause thyroid dysfunction because of the two iodine atoms two iodine atoms [22, 23]. It often causes an increase of T4 and rT3 and a decrease of T3 in serum that mainly related to the inhibition of 5'-deiodinase activity, resulting in a decrease in the production of T3 from T4 and a decrease in the clearance of rT3 [19–21]. In 14–18% of Amiodarone-treated patients, a thyroid dysfunction was observed that either related to Amiodarone-Induced Thyrothoxicosis (AIT) or Amiodarone -Induced Hypothyroidism (AIH) [24, 25]. Amiodarone also inhibits the peripheral conversion of thyroxine (T4) to triiodothyronine (T3) [21, 25]. At the extrathyroidal level, Amiodarone has the specific ability to inhibit 5′-monodeiodination of T4 [23]. Amiodarone causes changes in serum thyroxine (T4), triiodothyronine (T3), reverse triiodothyronine (rT3) and thyroid-stimulating hormone (TSH) concentrations. These changes are similar to those produced by iodinated radiographic contrast agents. The magnitude of these changes is dose dependent [24]. Amiodarone strongly inhibits type I, 5'-monodeiodinase enzyme activity that leads to changes in the rate of conversion of T4 to T3 [23, 24]. A decrease of 5′-deiodination of T4 to T3 is observed in many tissues but is most pronounced in the thyroid and the liver, the latter being the main extrathyroidal T3 production site [21]. This inhibitory action persists during and for several months after Amiodarone treatment, explaining the decreased plasma and tissue T3 concentrations [20, 21]. A decrease in T3 concentration affects the biological activity ensued by T3 hormone as T3 binds to its nuclear receptor that regulates many other cell biological activities [24–26]. The inhibition of type I 5'-deiodinase activity also results in the reduced clearance and a consequent rise in serum rT3 concentrations [23, 24]. Conversely, the inhibition of type II 5'-deiodinase activity by Amiodarone may lead to reduced intrapituitary T3 concentrations and this may in part account for the increase in serum TSH levels that was observed in patients treated with the drug [19–21]. AIH is believed to be the result of inability of the thyroid gland to escape from the Wolff-Chaikoff effect (according to Wolff-Chaikoff effect, the large amount of iodide that is released during the metabolism of Amiodarone leads to an adaptive blockage of further thyroidal iodide uptake and thyroid hormone biosynthesis). Furthermore, Amiodarone indirectly affects the thyroid hormone metabolism by inhibiting cellular thyroid hormone uptake. Results from kinetic studies suggested a decrease in the transfer of T4 from the plasma pool to rapidly exchangeable tissue pools, such as in the liver [21, 23], that leads to decreased availability of the substrate T4 intracellularly and hence reduced T3 production. A selective decrease in hepatic T4 transport was also demonstrated in hepatocytes and perfused rat liver as well as an impaired T3 uptake was observed in an anterior pituitary cell line [24, 25]. The risk of developing hypothyroidism is independent of the daily dose of Amiodarone. However, the risk is greater in the elderly and in female patients, probably as a result of a higher prevalence of underlying thyroid abnormality in this population [23, 25]. For example, it was shown that relative risk of developing AIH was 13-fold higher in female patients with positive thyroid thyroglobulin antibodies, as compared with men without thyroid antibodies [22, 23]. Another side effect of the drug is thyrotoxicosis which may occur anytime during therapy or even after the discontinuation of therapy. Hypothyroidism is usually an early event and it is uncommon after the first 18 months of Amiodarone treatment [22, 23]. AIH can be managed by either discontinuation of Amiodarone therapy or thyroid hormone replacement [19]. Although in some cases discontinuation of Amiodarone may not be feasible especially in the treatment of difficult ventricular tachyarrhythmia. In these cases, safer and more reliable option is thyroid hormone replacement therapy [23]. The following symptoms usually indicate the development of thyroid hypothyroidism which are associated with Amiodarone treatment, e.g. weight gain, cold intolerance, reduced physical activity and excessive bradycardia. The diagnosis is supported by a clear increase of TSH (thyroid stimulating hormone) in serum [21, 23]. Euthyroidism (normal level of thyroid hormone in serum) is usually should be obtained within 1–3 months following the discontinuation of treatment. AIT (Amiodarone- induced thyrotoxicosis) may occur during Amiodarone treatment or up to several months after discontinuation [26, 27]. AIT occurs in 2–12% of patients on chronic Amiodarone treatment. Clinical features in patients developing AIT such as weight loss, onset of arrhythmia, angina and congestive heart failure should alert the physician. The diagnosis is confirmed by a clear decrease in serum TSH level in which case Amiodarone should be withdrawn [23, 27]. Recovery from AIT usually occurs within a few months following drug withdrawal. There are two types of AIT. Type I is primarily related to excess iodine-induced thyroid hormone synthesis in an abnormal thyroid gland and Type II AIT which is developed by Amiodarone treatment is a destructive thyroiditis [28, 29]. In patients with preexisting thyroid abnormalities, thyrotoxicosis is believed to result from iodine-induced excessive thyroid hormone synthesis which is caused by drug treatment (Type I AIT) [29]. In this type of AIT, the pathogenesis is related to the effects of iodine overload by the drug on already abnormal thyroid glands, such as nodular goitre, autonomous nodule or latent Graves' disease [26, 27, 29]. However, in patients with an apparently normal thyroid gland, thyrotoxicosis results from the damage of thyroid gland by the drug that ensues the release of thyroid hormones into the circulation (Type II AIT) [27–29]. In vitro studies had shown Amiodarone to be cytotoxic to the thyroid cells; similarly, moderate to severe follicular damage and destruction were demonstrated in histopathological studies on thyroid gland tissues obtained from patients who were treated with the drug and showed symptoms of Type II AIT [26]. Clinical manifestations of AIT include palpitations, supraventicular tachycardia, weight loss, sweating and muscle weakness. By physical examination and ultra sonography of the thyroid the two types can be diagnosed and differentiated [22, 23, 30].

4.2. Pulmonary toxicity

There are numerous reports describing pulmonary toxicity associated with Amiodarone. Amiodarone-induced pulmonary toxicity (AIPT) occurs in 1–17% of patients. Acute pneumonitis and chronic fibrosis may be increased with higher circulating concentration of the drug [31, 32]. AIPT is more frequent in men and increases with age. Individuals with preexisting lung disease appear to be more susceptible to the drug [33, 34]. Pulmonary toxicity can be observed from the time of initiation of the treatment or after several years of treatment [32]. Regular x-ray of chest is recommended to be performed routinely in patients who are undergoing long-term therapy or when diagnosis is suspected. Once AIPT is diagnosed, treatment with corticosteroid and reduction or withdrawal of Amiodarone therapy should be carried out. Onset of dyspnoea or non-productive cough may be related to pulmonary toxicity such as interstitial pneumonitis [33–36]. In very rare cases when intravenous Amiodarone was administered, interstitial pneumonitis has been reported [35, 36]. Some of the symptoms of dyspnoea are fatigue, weight loss, and fever. Whether or not these symptoms are present in the patients, chest x-ray should be performed [34, 36]. In cases of development of interstitial pneumonitis in patients which is caused by Amiodarone therapy, early withdrawal of the drug is recommended. Symptoms usually resolve within 3–4 weeks followed by slow improvement in pulmonary function within several moths after withdrawal. Corticosteroid therapy expedites the recovery in these cases [32, 34]. In very rare cases severe respiratory complications sometimes fatal have been observed usually after surgery (Adult acute respiratory distress) [33, 35]. Amiodarone and its metabolite can cause lung damage by producing oxygen radicals and accumulation of phospholipids in the cells or by causing an immunological reaction [34, 35, 37]. The latter is supported by the finding of cytotoxic T cells in bronchoalveolar lavage fluid from patients who were diagnosed with AIPT [35]

A variety of recent studies suggest a critical role for alveolar cell apoptosis and lung fibrosis caused by the drug [34, 36]. We previously showed acute pathological changes including alveolar capillary congestion and infiltration of red blood cells into the lumen of alveoli in rabbits that were treated with the Amiodarone for two weeks [38]. Card also showed that the drug induces acute pulmonary inflammation following intratracheal administration of Amiodarone after 24 hours in a hamster model [39]. Electron microscopy of the lung tissues in Amiodarone treated rats showed pathological changes after three weeks [40]. These researchers showed the appearance of inclusion bodies inside the pneumocytes [40, 41]. One possible mechanism of lung damage by the drug is the accumulation of phosphlipids in the lung cells. The accumulation of inclusion bodies in the cytoplasm of the cells is thought to be due to decreased degradation of phospholipids because Amiodarone is a powerful inhibitor of degradation of phospholipids by lysosomes [38, 40, 41]. These inclusion bodies have also been detected in other tissues exposed to Amiodarone. Pitsiavas [40] found that Amiodarone induces specific ultrastructural changes in thyroid cells in rats. The specific changes included evidence of inclusion bodies and was also mentioned that Amiodarone is directly cytotoxic to the thyroid. There has also been debate in the past as to whether these inclusion bodies in cells in Amiodarone treated animals only reflect the ongoing cytotoxic process or whether these bodies are directly toxic to the cell in their own right. As mentioned earlier, Amiodarone causes the formation of inclusion bodies in many cell types. These changes are the result of inhibition of degradation of phospholipids by Amiodarone [40–42]. It has been shown that Amiodarone causes vacuolization in type II pneumocytes which are known as reactive type II pneumocytes [43]. The highest prevalence of reactive type II pneumocytes were noted in patients with systemic inflammatory response and alveolar hemorrhage [44–46]. In addition, reactive type II pneumocytes tended to occur more frequently in ventilator associated drug induced pulmonary disorders and they were associated mainly with the condition of acute lung injury [39, 44]. Microscopic observations showed diffused interstitial pneumonitis with widening of alveolar septa and interstitial fibrosis in lung tissues from patients [47, 48]. Organizing pneumonia, acute respiratory distress syndrome (ARDS), diffused alveolar hemorrhage (DAH) are the other adverse effects from Amiodarone administration [44, 47]. Interstitial pneumonitis is the most common adverse effect of Amiodarone which presents after two months of therapy with 400 mg per day [35]. The symptoms are fever, cough, pleuritic pain and weight loss. Accumulated phospholipids in lung cells because of drug treatment, interfere with metabolism of cells which results cell injury and death [35, 44]. Alteration of the phospholipids of cellular and organelle membrane by Amiodarone leads to change in their functions [35, 41, 42]. Angiotensin enzyme increases Amiodarone-induced lung toxicity [36, 45, 47]. Other pulmonary side effects from Amiodarone treatment include fibrosis that is the result of chronic inflammation which in turn is due to cellular damage, reduced forced vital capacity, total lung capacity and reduced diffusing capacity. Other Amiodarone side effect on lung is organizing pneumonia which is accompanied with the proliferation of granulation tissue which consists of fibroblasts, myofibroblast and collagen fibers [35, 45, 48]. Acute respiratory distress syndrome (ARDS) is characterized by diffuse alveolar hemorrhage which includes pulmonary edema, systemic lupus vasculitis and hemorrhage [35]. The more common form AIPT is associated with doses of 400 mg daily or more. AIPT is reversible if diagnosed early [31, 49].

http://dx.doi.org/10.5772/60418

4.3. Cardiac toxicity

Amiodarone by blocking the calcium channel activity can cause sinus bradycardia and AV nodal block in 5% of patients. Hypotension may occur when concentrated Amiodarone hydrochloride injection is given by the intravenous route. In some cases, hypotension may be refractory, resulting in fatal outcomes [8, 18].

4.4. Hepatotoxicity

Hepatptoxicity is common with higher doses of Amiodarone. Elevation of serum enzymes are reported in 15–50% of patients in long-term therapy. Regular monitoring of liver function tests (measuring of serum aspartate aminotransaminases, serum alanine aminotransferase glutamyl transepeptidase levels) is recommended as soon as Amiodarone treatment is started and during the treatment. The elevation of these enzymes is usually asymptomatic. These changes are dependent on the dose of the drug. Acute liver disorders including severe hepatocellular insufficiency or hepatic failure, sometimes fatal and chronic liver disorders may occur with oral and intravenous forms within the first 24 hours of i.v. Amiodarone [50, 51]. Therefore, Amiodarone dose should be reduced or the treatment discontinued if the transaminases increase exceeds three times the normal range [51, 52]. Because of the potential risk of hepatotoxicity and/or accumulation, Amiodarone should be used with extreme caution in patients with hepatic disease [50, 51]. Histologic examination of biopsy samples from Amiodarone-induced cirrhotic patients showed that drug-induced cirrhosis is similar to alcoholic cirrhosis. Close examination of liver tissues from the patients showed leukocytic infiltrate and strikingly high Mallory's hyaline along with other usual pathologic findings of cirrhosis are noted [53–55]. Mallory's hyaline is an eosinophilic inclusion made up of intermediate keratin filaments. Mallory's hyaline can be seen in primary biliary cirrhosis, alcoholic cirrhosis or hepatitis, nonalcoholic cirrhosis and some other conditions [50, 52]. Other histological evidences revealed accumulation of granules in macrophages, intralobular inflammatory infiltrates, fibrosis and phospholipidosis. Electron microscopy observation shows abnormal mitochondria and phospholipid laden lysosomes [53, 54]. Amiodarone causes direct damage to membrane lipid bilayer and changes in mitochondrial function. Amiodarone as a potent inhibitor of phospholipase A that promotes the accumulation of lipid rich materials in lysosomes. The studies showed that mitochondrial dysfunction leads to fibrosis. Patients with hepatotoxicity from Amiodarone have symptoms such as fatigue, nausea, weight loss, hepatomegaly, elevation of serum aminotransferase and alkaline phosphate levels [55, 56].

4.5. The effects of Amiodarone on ocular tissue

Corneal deposits develop in almost all patients and regular ophthalmological monitoring (e.g. slit lamp biomicroscopy, visual acuity, ophthalmoscopy, etc.) is recommended. If blurred or decreased vision occurs, ophthalmological examination including fundoscopy should be promptly performed. Appearance of optic neuropathy and/or optic neuritis requires Amiodarone withdrawal due to the potential progression to blindness [57, 58]. Electron microscopic observation revealed the presence of lysosomal-like intracytoplasmic membranous lamellar bodies in extraocular muscle fibers, corneal epithelium, stromal and endothelial cells, conjunctival epithelium, scleral cells, lens epithelium, iris, ciliary body, choroid, retinal pigment epithelium, ganglion cells, large diameter axons of the optic nerve, the endothelium of ocular blood vessels and basal cells of corneal epithelium. Lamellar bodies in these cells contained iodine [53, 59]. Deposits were observed in the corneal epithelium of Amiodarone treated patients [59] about one week after the initiation of treatment with Amiodarone [59], keratopathy, unilateral and bilateral anterior ischemic optic neuropathy are also occurred [60, 61]. The corneal deposits are caused by secretion of Amiodarone from lacrimal gland on corneal surface. These deposits are brown and have been described as resembling cat's whiskers [57, 58]. Amiodarone- induced ocular side effects are time and dose-dependent. The changes are reversible after stopping Amiodarone treatment. Amiodarone-related optic neuropathy has been reported after 4 month duration of treatment with unilateral or bilateral visual loss that can progress to blindness [62, 63]. Microscopic studies showed the accumulation of lamellar inclusions in the axons of the optic nerve because of drug induced lipidosis [57, 63].

5. Other side effects of Amiodarone

Dermatologic, gastrointestinal, neurologic and genitourinary changes are the other side effects of chronic use of Amiodarone. Photosensitivity and less frequently phototoxicity are important dermatological side effects. Photosensitivity is quite common and there is a wide spectrum of skin reactions, ranging from an increased propensity to suntan to intense burning and erythema and swelling of the exposed area [64, 65]. Phototoxicity induces blue-gray skin hyperpigmentation of predominantly sun exposed areas. It develops in <10% of patients, preferentially affecting men. It was mainly observed after an average of 20 months of continuous Amiodarone treatment and a minimal cumulative dose of 160 g [64, 66]. Histopathologically, Amiodarone-induced phototoxicity has been related to lysosomal dermal lipofuscin deposits. The only treatment is reduction or cessation of therapy, upon which skin changes may slowly abate [64, 66]. However, skin discoloration is likely to persist for years. The intensity of these reactions could be alleviated by a reduction in dosage or by application of a protective sunscreen. Patients should be instructed to avoid exposure to the sun or use protective measures during therapy [64–66].

Peripheral neuropathy has been observed in 3–30% of patients on long-term high dosage (generally over 400mg/day) regimen which include tremor, ataxia and sleep disturbances. Histologically, inclusion bodies and segmental demyelination of the nerve fibers have been demonstrated in peripheral nerve fibers. After discontinuation of the medicine, the neurological complication is slowly and incompletely resolved [65, 67].

A significant association was found between the development of epididymitis and high-dose Amiodarone treatment for a long time. Genitourinary effects include sterile epididymitis with pain and swelling in the scrotum [68].

6. Conclusion

Side effects occur more frequently with long-term administration of the drug, e.g. more than 6 months and is related to total dose of the drug administered; therefore the effectiveness of Amiodarone in long-term treatment of patients with heart arrhythmia is limited because of the development of its adverse side effects.

Author details

Fereshteh Mehraein[1,2]

Address all correspondence to: femehra@yahoo.com

1 Anatomy Department, Faculty of Medicine, Iran University of Medical Sciences, Tehran, Iran

2 Minimally Invasive Surgery Research Center, Iran University of Medical Sciences, Tehran, Iran

References

[1] Vaughan Williams EM. Classification of anti-arrhythmic drugs:In: Sandoe E, Flensted-Jensen E, Olesen KII, eds. Symposium on Cardiac Arrhythmias, Stockholm, Sweden, Astra. 1970;449–472.

[2] Siddoway LA. Pharmacologic principals of antiarrhythmic drugs.In: Podrid PJ, Kowey PR:eds. Cardiac arrhythmia: Mechanisms, diagnosis, and management. Baltimore, Md: Williams & Wilkins;1995.

[3] Bigger JT Jr. Antiarrhythmic treatment: an overview. Am J Cardiol. :1984;5:8B–16B.

[4] Chung S, Reinier K, Teodorescu C, Evanado A, Kehr E, Al Samara M, et al. Epidemiology of sudden cardiac death: clinical and research progress in cardiovascular disease. Prog Cardiovasc Dis.2008;51(3):213–28.

[5] Wiener N, Rosenblueth A. The mathematical formulation of the problem of conduction of impulses in a network of connected excitable elements, specifically in cardiac muscle. Archives del instituto de cardiologia de Mexico.1946;16(3):205–65.

[6] Plomp TA. Analytical profiles of Amiodarone in analytical profiles of drug substances. San Diego. K Florey ed. Academic Press Inc., 1991.

[7] Deltour G, Binon F, Tondeur R, Goldenberg C, Henaux F, Sion R, et al. Studies in the benzofuran series.VI. Coronary – dilating activity of alkylated and aminoalkylated derivatives of 3-benzoylbenzofuran. Arch Int Pharmacodyn Ther:1962;139:247–54.

[8] Goldschlager N, Epstein AE, Naccarelli G, Olshansky B, Singh B. Practical guidelines for clinicians who treat patients with Amiodarone. Practice Guidelines Subcommittee, North American Society of Pacing and Electrophysiology. Arch Intern Med. 2000;160:1741–8.

[9] Vassalo P, Trhman RG. Prescribing Amiodarone. JAMA:2007;298:1312–22.

[10] Scheinman MM, Levine JH, Cannom DS, Friehling T, Kopelman HA, Chilson DA, et al. Dose-ranging study of intravenous Amiodarone in patients with life-threatening ventricular tachyarrhythmias. The Intravenous Amiodarone Multicenter Investigators Group. Circulation. 1995;92(11):3264.

[11] Siddoway L. Amiodarone: Guidelines for use and monitoring. Am Fam Physician. 2003;68:2189–96.

[12] Podrid PJ. Amiodarone: Reevaluation of an old drug. Ann Intern Med.1995;122:689–700.

[13] Primeau R, Agh A, Giorgi C. Long term efficacy and toxicity of Amiodarone in the treatment of refractory cardiac arrhythmias. Can J Cardiol:1989;5:98–104.

[14] Zimetbaum P. Amiodarone for atrial fibrillation. N Eng J Med. 2007;356:935–41.

[15] Rosenbaum MB, Chiale PA, Halpern MS, Nau GT, Przybylski J, Levi RJ, et al: Clinical efficacy of Amiodarone as an anti-arrhythmic agent. Am J Cardiol.1976; 38: 934.

[16] Connolly SJ. Evidence-based analysis of Amiodarone efficacy and safety. Circulation. 1999;100(19):2025.

[17] Desai AD, Chun S, Sung RJ. The role of intravenous Amiodarone in the management of cardiac arrhythmias. Ann Intern Med.1997;127(4):294.

[18] Vorperian VR, Havighurst TC, Miller S, January CT. Adverse effects of low dose Amiodarone: a meta-analysis. J Am Coll Cardiol:1997;30(3):791.

[19] Harjai KJ, Licata AA. Effects of Amiodarone on thyroid function. Ann Intern Med. 1997;126:63–73.

[20] Lambert MJ, Burger G, Galeazzi RL, Engler D. Are selective increases in serum thyroxine (T4) due to iodinated inhibitor for T4 monodeiodination indicative of hyperthyroidism? J Clin Endocrinol Metab.1982;55:1058–65.

[21] Kennedy RL, Griffiths H, Gray TA. Amiodarone and the thyroid. Clin Chem. 1989;35:1882–7.

[22] Newman CM, Price A, Davis DW, Gray TA, Weetman AP. Amiodarone and the thyroid: a practice guide to the management of thyroid dysfunction induced by Amiodarone therapy.Heart.1998;79:121–7.

[23] Figge HL, Figge J. The effects of Amiodarone on thyroid hormone function: a review of physiology and clinical manifestations. J Clin Pharmacol.1990;30:588–95.

[24] Martino E, Bartalena L, Mariotti S, Aghini-Lombardi F, Ceccarelli C, Lippi F, et al. Radioactive iodine thyroid uptake in patients with Amiodarone-iodine-induced thyroid dysfunction. Acta Endocrinol 1988;119:167–73.

[25] Harjai KJ, Licata AA. Effects of Amiodarone on thyroid function. Ann Intern Med 1997;126:63– 73.

[26] Brennan MD, Erickson DZ, Carney JA, Bahn, RS. Nongoitrous Amiodarone-associated thyrotoxicosis: evidence of follicular disruption in vitro and in vivo. Thyroid. 1995;5:177–83.

[27] Bartalena L, Brogioni S, Grasso L, Bogazzi F, Burelli A, Martino E. Treatment of Amiodarone-induced thyrotoxicosis, a difficult challenge: results of a prospective study. J Clin Endocrinol Metab. 1996;81:2930–3.

[28] Cappiello E, Boldorini R, Tosoni A, Piraneo S, Bernasconi R, Raggi U. Ultrastructural evidence of thyroid damage in Amiodarone-induced thyrotoxicosis. J Endocrinol Invest.1995;18:862–8.

[29] Tsang W, Houlden RL. Amiodarone induced thyrotoxicosis:A review. Can J Cardiol: 2009;25(7):421–4.

[30] Rormensch HH, Belhassen B, Swanson BN, Shoshani D, Spielman SR, Greenspon AJ, et al. Steady-state serum Amiodarone concentrations: Relationship with antiarrhythmic efficacy and toxicity. Ann Intern Med.1984;101:462–9.

[31] Ernawati DF, Stafford L, Hughes FD. Amiodarone Induced pulmonary toxicity. BR J Clin Pharmacol.2008;66:82–7.

[32] Kudenchuk PJ, Pierson DJ, Greene HL, Graham EL, Sears GK, Troubaugh GB: prospective evaluation of Amiodarone pulmonary toxicity. Chest.1984;86:541–548.

[33] Camus P, Martin WJ, II, Rosenow EC, III. Amiodarone pulmonary toxicity. Clin Chest Med.2004;25:65–75.

[34] Martin WJ, Rosenow EC. Amiodarone pulmonary toxicity: Recognition and pathogenesis (part:2). Chest.1988;93:1242–8.

[35] Wolkove N, Baltzan M. Amiodarone pulmonary toxicity. Can respir J: 2009;16(2):43–48.

[36] Uhal BD, Wang R, Laukka J, et al. Inhibition of Amiodarone induced lung fibrosis but not alveolitis by angiotensin system antagonists. Basic Clin Phrmacol Toxicol. Feb 2003;92(2):81–87.

[37] Verchei A, Blazovics A, Gyorgy I, Feher E, Toth M, Szenasi G, et al. The role of free radicals in the pathogenesis of Amiodarone toxicity. J Cardovasc Electrophysiol: 1993;4:161–177.

[38] Mehraein F, Shams A. Amiodarone induced morphological changes in rabbit pneumocytes. Yakhteh Medical Journal:2009, 11(1):13–16.

[39] Card JW, Raz WJ, Brien JF, Margolin SB, Massey TE. Differential effects of pirferridone on acute pulmonary injury and ensuing fibrosis in the hamster model of Amiodarone induced pulmonary toxicity. Toxicol Sci:2003, 75:169–180.

[40] Pitsiavas V, Smerdely P, Li M, Boyages SC.Amiodarone induces a different pattern of ultrastructural changes in the thyroid to iodine excess alone in both the BB/W rat and the Wistar rat. Eur J Endocrinol:1997;137:89–98.

[41] Bartussio A, Marzini S. Agostini M, Alberti A, Cimenti C, Bruttomesso D, et al. Amiodarone inhibits lung degradation of SPA and perturbs the distribution of lysosomal enzymes. AM J Physiol Lung Cell Mol Physiol:2001;281:l1189–99.

[42] Hruban Z. Pulmonary and generalized lysosomal storage induced by amphiphilic drugs. Environ Health Prospect. 1984;33:53–76.

[43] Linsson K, Jacobe J, Poletti VE, van Mook W, Cornelissen EL. Reactive typeII pneumocytes in bronchoalveolar lavage fluid. Acta Cytol:2004;48:497–504.

[44] Marchlinski FE, Gansler TS, Waxman HL, Josephson ME. Amiodarone pulmonary toxicity. Ann Int Med.1982;97:839–45.

[45] Ashrafian H, Davey P. Is Amiodarone an underrecognized cause of acute respiratory failure in the ICU. Chest. 2001;120:275–82.

[46] Iskandar SB, Abi-saleh B, Keith RL, Byrd RP Jr, Roy TM. Amiodarone-induced alveolar hemorrhage. South Med J. 2006;99:329–30.

[47] Ott MC, Khoor A, Leventhal JP, Paterick TE, Burger CD. Pulmonary toxicity in patients receiving low-dose Amiodarone. Chest. 2006;123:646–51.

[48] Seki S, Itagaki S, Kobayashi M, Hirano T, Iseki K. Amiodarone increases the accumulation of DEA in a human alveolar epithelium derived cell line. Biol Pharm Bull. 2008;31:1449.

[49] Larsen BT, Vaszar LT, Colby TV, Tazelaar HD. Lymphoid hyperplasia and eosinophilic pneumonia as histologic manifestations of amiodarone induced lung toxicity. Am J Surg Pathol.2012;36:509.

[50] Lewis JH, Mullick F, Ishak KG, Ranard RC, Raqsdale B, Perse RM.et al. Histopathologic analysis of suspected amiodarone hepatotoxicity. Hum Pathol:1990; 21: 59–67.

[51] Ioannou GN, Boyko EJ, Lee SP. The prevalence and predictors of elevated serum aminotransferase activity in the United States in 1999–2002. Am J Gastroenterol. 2006; 101: 76–82.

[52] Lewis H, Ranard RC, Caruso A, Jackson LK, Mullick F, Ishak KG.et al., Amiodarone hepatotoxicity: prevalence and clinicopathologic correlations among 104 patients. Hepatology. 1989 ;9(5):679–685.

[53] Puli SR, Fraley MA, Puli V, Kuperman AB, Poucell S, Ireton J, et al. Amiodarone-associated phospholipidosis and fibrosis of the liver: light immunohistochemical and electron microscopic studies. Gastroenterology. 1984;86(5 Pt 1):926.

[54] Alpert MA. Hepatic cirrhosis caused by low-dose oral Amiodarone therapy. Am J Med Sci. 2005;330(5):257–261.

[55] Simon JB, Manley PN, Brien JF, Armstrong PW. Amiodarone hepatotoxicity simulating alcoholic liver disease. N Engl J Med. 1984; 311: 167–172.

[56] Pollak PT, Shafer SL. Use of population modeling to define rational monitoring of Amiodarone hepatic effects. Clin Pharmacol Ther. 2004; 75: 342–351.

[57] 57:Mäntyjärvi M, Tuppurainen K, Ikäheimo K. Ocular side effects of Amiodarone. Surv Ophthalmol: 1998;42(4):360.

[58] Ingram DV. Ocular effects in long-term Amiodarone therapy. Am Heart J. 1983;106(4 Pt 2):902.

[59] Haug SJ, Friedman AH: Identification of Amiodarone in corneal deposits. Am J Ophthalmol: 1991;111:518–19.

[60] Kaplan LJ, Cappaert WE: Amiodarone keratopathy. correlation to dosage and duration. Arch Ophthalmol.1982; 100:601–2.

[61] Flach AJ, Dolan BJ. Progression of Amiodarone induced cataracts. Doc Ophthalmol: 1993;83:323.

[62] Thystrup JD, Fledelius HC: Retinal maculopathy possibly associated with Amiodarone medication. Acta Ophthalmol:1994; 72:639–641.

[63] Macaluso DC, Shults WT, Fraunfelder FT. Features of Amiodarone- induced optic neuropathy. Am J Ophtalmol:1999;127:610.

[64] Enseleit F, Wyss CA, Duru F, Noll G, Ruschitzka F. Images in cardiovascular medicine. The blue man: Amiodarone-induced skin discoloration. Circulation. 2006;113(5):e63.

[65] Vrobel TR, Miller PE, Mostow ND, Rakita L: A general overview of Amiodarone toxicity: its prevention, detection, and management. Prog Cardiovasc Dis. 1989;31:393–426.

[66] Kounis NG, Frangides C, Papadaki PJ, Zavras GM, Goudevenos J. Dose-dependent appearance and disappearance of Amiodarone-induced skin pigmentation. Clin Cardiol. 1996;19(7):592.

[67] Orr CF, Ahlskog JE. Frequency, characteristics, and risk factors for Amiodarone neurotoxicity.Arch Neurol. 2009;66(7):865.

[68] Ibsen HHW, Frandsen F, Brandrup F, Moller M. Epididymitis caused by treatment with Amiodarone.Genitourin Med. 1989;65:257–258.